AF364432

PHARMACEUTICS-I
(GENERAL PHARMACY)
A Practical Manual

PHARMACEUTICS-I
(GENERAL PHARMACY)
A Practical Manual

N. K. Jain

M. Pharm., Ph.D., LL.M., FIC
Professor of Pharmaceutics
Department of Pharmaceutical Sciences,
Dr. H. S. Gour (Central) University,
Sagar- 470003 (MP).

Vijay Mishra

M. Pharm.
Department of Pharmaceutical Sciences,
Dr. H. S. Gour (Central) University,
Sagar- 470003 (MP).

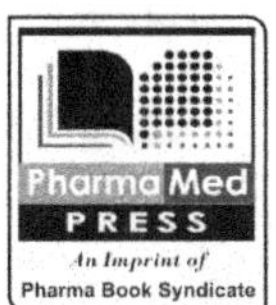

PharmaMed Press

An imprint of Pharma Book Syndicate

A unit of BSP Books Pvt. Ltd.

4-4-309/316, Giriraj Lane,

Sultan Bazar, Hyderabad - 500 095.

© 2012, *by Publisher*
Fourth Reprint 2019

All rights reserved. No part of this book or parts thereof may be reproduced, stored in a retrieval system or transmitted in any language or by any means, electronic, mechanical, photocopying, recording or otherwise without the prior written permission of the publishers.

Published by

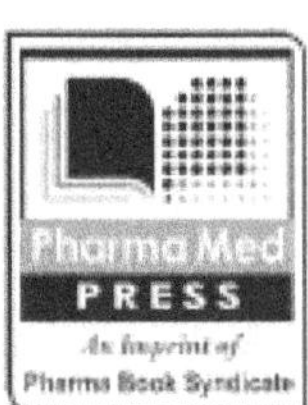

PharmaMed Press

An imprint of Pharma Book Syndicate

A unit of BSP Books Pvt. Ltd.

4-4-309/316, Giriraj Lane, Sultan Bazar, Hyderabad - 500 095.

Phone: 040-23445600, 23445688; Fax: 91+40-23445611

E-mail: info@pharmamedpress.com

www.pharmamedpress.com/pharmamedpress.net

ISBN: 978-93-89974-88-1

PREFACE

General Pharmacy is the foundation of pharmaceutics knowledge to students entering into pharmaceutical profession. Although several books covering the theoretical aspects of General Pharmacy exclusively are now available yet a manual explaining the practical as well as the theoretical aspects are not available so far. This practical manual has been framed keeping in view the new and revised syllabus as prescribed by different universities of India like Gautam Buddh Technical University (GBTU), Lucknow; Rajeev Gandhi Technical University (RGPV), Bhopal; Jawaharlal Nehru Technology University, Hyderabad and many other universities.

This manual has been written in a very simple language to make pharmacy students to understand the topics related to preparation of various dosage forms in a simplified manner.

This practical manual includes 22 Chapters and 34 Exercises comprising 131 preparations covering the topics prescribed in the syllabus. The topics covered are Aromatic Waters, Solutions, Syrups, Elixirs, Spirits, Powders, Lotions, Liniments, Mucilage, Glycerins, Inhalation, Tinctures and Extracts, Pastes, Jellies, Ear Preparations, Eye Preparations, Nasal Preparations, Pills, Lozenges, Pastilles, as well as Exercises on Size Reduction and Solid-Solid Mixing.

Each chapter contains informative notes on particular dosage forms like introductory information, methods of preparation, therapeutic uses, dose, storage conditions, specific labeling requirement, contraindication (if any), marketed preparations and specimen label.

For further improvement of subsequent editions of this book, any suggestions, criticism and comments both from students and teachers will be greatly appreciated.

Dec 2011

Sagar

- Authors

Contents

CHAPTER 5

Exercise 10

CHAPTER 6

Exercise 11

Exercise 12

CHAPTER 7

CHAPTER 10

Exercise 18

CHAPTER 11

Exercise 19

CHAPTER 12

CHAPTER 21
SIZE REDUCTION

Exercise 33

CHAPTER 22
MIXING OF SOLIDS

Exercise 34

CHAPTER 1

AROMATIC WATERS

The British Pharmacopoeia (BP) defines aromatic waters are clear, saturated aqueous solutions of volatile oils or other aromatic or volatile substances.

Aromatic waters are saturated solutions (unless otherwise specified) of volatile oils (c.g. Rose oil, peppermint oil) or other aromatic or volatile substances, e.g. Camphor in purified water. Aromatic waters are prepared from a number of volatile substances, including peppermint oil, rose oil, orange flower oil, spearmint oil, anise oil, wintergreen oil, camphor and chloroform. Naturally, they possess an odor and taste similar to that plant or volatile substance from which they are prepared. Aromatic waters are clear and free from solid impurities and are free from empyreumatic (smoke like) or foreign odors. Most of the aromatic substances in the preparation of aromatic waters have very low solubility in water and even though water may be saturated, its concentration of aromatic material is still rather small. The volatile substances from which the aromatic waters are to be prepared should be of purest quality.

Aromatic waters can be categorized in two types as-

1. **Simple aromatic waters:** They contain purified water as a solvent but do not contain alcohol and are mainly used as vehicles e.g. Chloroform water.

2. **Concentrated aromatic waters:** They contain alcohol as solvent for the volatile constituents. Examples of concentrated aromatic waters are Camphor Water BP, Concentrated Peppermint Water BP, Concentrated Caraway Water BPC, Concentrated Cinnamon Water BPC, Concentrated Dill Water BPC, Concentrated Anise Water BPC etc.

Methods of Preparation

Aromatic waters may be prepared by distillation or solution of the aromatic substance, with or without the use of dispersing agents.

1. Distillation Method

The distillation method involves the placing of the coarsely ground odoriferous portion of the plant or drug from which the aromatic water is to be prepared in a suitable still, with sufficient purified water. Most of the volume of water is then distilled. The excess oil collected with the distillate rises to the top of the aqueous product and is removed. The remaining aqueous solution, saturated with volatile material requires clarification by filtration. This is the common method of preparation of aromatic waters although it is slow and expensive one, e.g. Strong Rose Water NF and Orange Flower Water NF are prepared by this method. These waters have active volatile constituents in small quantities so it may be necessary to repeat the distillation process several times.

2. Solution Method

This method is simpler, quicker and more economical as compared to distillation method. In this method, aromatic water is prepared by intermittently shaking 2 ml (if liquid) or 2 g (if solid) of the volatile substance with 1000 ml of purified water in suitable container for a period of 15 minutes. After the period of agitation the mixture is set aside for 12 hours or longer to permit the excess oil and the solid substance to settle. Without further agitation the mixture is passed through a wetted filter paper and purified water added as needed to bring the volume of the filtrate up to the prescribed quantity.

3. Alternative Solution Method

By this method, the volatile oil or suitably comminuted aromatic solid is thoroughly incorporated with 15 g of powdered talc or a sufficient quantity of kieselghur or pulp filter paper and to this mixture is added 1000 ml of purified water. The resulting slurry is thoroughly agitated several times for the period of 30 minutes and then filtered. Powdered talc, kieselghur and pulp filter paper work as filter aid which renders the formulation more clear and also as distributing agents for the aromatic substances that ultimately increases the surface area of aromatic substances exposed to the solvent action of water. The distributing agents should be inert in nature.

Preparation of Concentrated Aromatic Water

These products are alcoholic, non aqueous preparations containing 2% of volatile oils. They are 40 times stronger than the ordinary aromatic waters. Many volatile oils contain aromatic part and non-aromatic part. The aromatic portion is much more soluble in a weak alcohol than the non-aromatic portion. Hence when a solution of the oil in 90% alcohol is diluted with a limited amount of water the aromatic portion of the oil remains in solution while the non-aromatic portion is precipitated off, separating as an oily layer. Therefore 50 g of talc is added for 1000 ml of preparation, which acts as a distributing agent, and will absorb the non-aromatic part. The solution is agitated and set aside for a few hours and filtered.

Therapeutic Uses

Aromatic waters are pharmaceutical aid and used principally for perfuming and flavoring the formulation. They can be used as an excipients or bases or vehicles for formulation of other pharmaceutical preparations. Aromatic waters may be used for some special purposes like,

(a) Camphor water has been used as the vehicle in ophthalmic solutions owning to its ability to contribute refreshing and stimulating effect to the preparation.

(b) Rose water has an antioxidant activity. The Rose water cleanses, tones and protects skin from harmful environmental impacts.

(c) Hamamelis water known as witch hazel is employed as a rub, perfume and as an astringent in various cosmetic preparations, particularly in after-shave lotions.

(d) Chloroform water has been used as preservative apart from its flavoring nature.

Dose

The dose of simple aromatic waters is usually 15 to 30 ml but varies from water to water.

Storage Conditions

Aromatic waters deteriorate with time and hence should be made in small quantities and protected from intense light and excessive heat. They should be stored in airtight, light resistance container in cool place.

Aromatic waters should be protected from strong light and preferably stored in containers which are stoppered with purified cotton to allow access of some air but to exclude dust.

Specific Labeling Requirement

The label should have the caution 'PROTECT FROM SUN LIGHT' with red ink due to the presence of volatile constituent in the preparation. This caution is more important in case of Chloroform water as chloroform gets converted into poisonous phosgene gas.

Examples of Aromatic Waters

1. Chloroform Water BP

Composition	Method of Preparation	Caution
1. Double-strength chloroform water- Chloroform- 0.5 ml Purified water q.s.-100 ml **2. Concentrated chloroform water-** Chloroform-10 ml Ethanol- q.s. Purified water q.s.-100 ml	Chloroform water can be prepared simply by adding chloroform (2.5 ml) to purified water (1000 ml) and shaking frequently until the chloroform is in solution. For double strength chloroform water, one part of the concentrated chloroform water should be diluted with 19 parts of purified water (1 in 20 dilutions); this must be further diluted 1:1 to produce a product with a final chloroform content of 0.25% v/v. To produce a solution having an equivalent strength to chloroform water, one part of concentrated chloroform water should be diluted with 39 parts of purified water (1 in 40 dilutions).	In preparations having a high content of dissolved solids a lower concentration (0.15% v/v) may be necessary to avoid problems with "salting out" of the chloroform. Further chloroform forms harmful phosgene gas in presence of light.

Label

CHLOROFORM WATER BP **(50 ml)**		
Composition: Each 50 ml contains, Chloroform- 0.125 ml Purified water q.s.- 50 ml **Dose:** 15 to 30 ml **Storage:** Store in airtight, light-resistant container in cool place.	**CHLORWATER** (Aromatic Water) (Used for perfuming, flavoring the formulation, as vehicle and also as a preservative at 25% v/v) **PROTECT FROM SUN LIGHT** **NOT FOR INJECTION**	**Mfg. Lic. No.-** 2V/2010 **Batch No.-** YM 0512 **Mfg. Date-** Mar. 2011 **Exp. Date-** Feb. 2012 **M.R.P.-** Rs. 15.00 (Inclusive of all taxes) **Mfd. By:** YAVI PHARMA KANPUR ROAD, LUCKNOW UP- 226001

2. Camphor Water BP; USP

Camphor [$C_{10}H_{16}O$], is a ketone or a keto-tetrahydro-cymene, obtained from the camphor tree, *Cinnamomum camphora.*

Composition	Method of Preparation	Caution
1. Camphor Water BP- Camphor- 1 part Purified Water q.s.- 1000 parts **2. Concentrated Camphor Water BP-** Camphor- 40 g Alcohol (90%)- 600 ml Purified water q.s.- 1000 ml **3. Camphor Water USP-** Camphor- 8 g Alcohol- 5 ml Precipitated calcium phosphate- 5 g Distilled water q.s.- 1000 ml	Camphor is triturated with alcohol and precipitated calcium phosphate, water is added gradually and filtered. The first trituration with alcohol, renders it more readily pulverizable by destroying the tenacity with which the particles of camphor adhere together, the second trituration with the calcium salt subdivides it still more finely, so that the water can more readily act upon it, and produce the desired medicated water. The filtration removes the calcium phosphate and excess of camphor from the solution. **Note-** Ice-cold water will dissolve more camphor than water at the ordinary temperature.	Purified water should not be added to the alcoholic solution of camphor because doing this whole of the camphor will be precipitated out which will not redissolve easily on shaking.

Label

CAMPHOR WATER USP (50 ml)		
Composition: Each 50 ml contains, Camphor- 0.4 g Ethanol (90 %)- 0.25 ml Distilled water q.s.- 50 ml **Dose:** 30 to 60 ml **Storage:** Store in airtight, light-resistant container in cool place to prevent the volatilization of camphor.	**CAMPWATER** (Aromatic Water) (Flavoring agent, mild carminative in flatulence, diaphoretic, expectorant and as an antiseptic for the alimentary canal) **PROTECT FROM SUN LIGHT** **NOT FOR INJECTION**	**Mfg. Lic. No.-** 5D/2010 **Batch No.-** AK 0502 **Mfg. Date-** Jun. 2011 **Exp. Date-** May. 2012 **M.R.P.-** Rs. 20.00 (Inclusive of all taxes) **Mfd. By:** YAVI PHARMA KANPUR ROAD, LUCKNOW UP- 226001

It mildly excites the circulation, dilating the superficial vessels and slightly increasing the cardiac output. It also directly excites cerebrum. It is also used for its calming influence in hysteria, nervousness, neuralgia and for serious diarrhea.When applied externally, camphor dilates the vessels of the skin, and is used as a rubefacient and mild counter-irritant in rheumatisms, sprains bronchitis and in inflammatory conditions. Campor has great value in colds, chills, and in all inflammatory complaints.

Camphor is present in several over-the-counter (OTC) compounds and therefore may be ingested by small children. Because seizures may follow ingestion of certain amounts, so appropriate treatment is needed, including the use of anticonvulsant.

3. Rose Water USP/NF

Rose water was first obtained by distilling roses in Persia (Iran). Rose perfumes are made from attar of roses or rose oil, which is a mixture of volatile essential oils, obtained by steam-distilling the crushed petals of roses. Rose water is the hydrosol portion of the distillate of rose petals. Rose water is simply water that has been flavored with roses by distillation of rose petals.

The unexpanded petals are plucked as a whole from the calyx, and the lighter-colored basal portions cut off. They are used both fresh and dried; in the latter case being gently sifted to remove any stamens. The petals generally occur in little conical masses, easily separated into the individual petals, which are obcordate in shape, velvety and of a deep purplish-red color. They possess a delicate, rose-like aroma, and a slightly astringent taste.

Rose water can be prepared from Rose (*Rosa centifolia,* Family- Rosaceae) flowers by distillation method.

Rose water is colorless, clear, strong, pleasant odor and taste of fresh rose blossoms, free from empyreuma, mustiness or fungi growths; neutral or slightly acidic.

Rose water has antioxidant activity. Extract of the rose is capable of relieving skin ailments caused by circulation problems. It can reduce the redness and improve the general condition of the skin. It is suitable for all skin types. Rose water also is useful for hair. It makes hair glossy and healthy looking. It is a constituent of *Mistura Ferri Composita*, and is used as a flavoring agent in the preparation of the BP Rose basis for lozenges. Rose water has a very distinctive flavor and is also used for religious purposes.

Rose water is better known as an ingredient in cosmetics than as food flavoring. The official Rose Water Ointment NF formulation was developed by Galen. It should be diluted with twice its volume of distilled water immediately before use, unless otherwise specified.

Composition	Method of Preparation
Rose oil- 2 ml Ethanol (90 %)- 2 ml Purified water q.s.- 100 ml	Rose Water is prepared by mixing rose oil (2 ml) and ethanol (2 ml) then make up the volume 100 ml with purified water. Rose Water USP is prepared by mixing equal volumes of Stronger Rose Water and distilled water. Stronger Rose Water (Aqua Rosae Fortior, USP) is obtained by distilling the flowers of *Rosa damascene* (Family- Rosaceae).

Label

ROSE WATER NF (50 ml)		
Composition: Each 50 ml contains, Rose oil- 1 ml Ethanol (90 %)- 1 ml Purified water q.s.- 50 ml **Dose:** 8 to 30 ml **Storage:** Store in airtight, light-resistant container in cool place.	**ROSE SHINE** (Aromatic Water) (Flavoring agent, mild carminative, diaphoretic, for skin ailments, used in lotions for its fragrant odor and as a mild astringent) **PROTECT FROM SUN LIGHT** **NOT FOR INJECTION**	**Mfg. Lic. No.-** 2J/2010 **Batch No.-** VD 0311 **Mfg. Date-** Aug. 2011 **Exp. Date-** July 2012 **M.R.P.-** Rs. 35.00 (Inclusive of all taxes) **Mfd. By:** YAVI PHARMA KANPUR ROAD, LUCKNOW UP- 226001

4. Peppermint Water USP

Peppermint oil is extracted from *Mentha piperita* (Family- Labiatae). The main chemical components of peppermint oil are menthol, menthone, 1,8-cineole, methyl acetate, methofuran, isomenthone, limonene, β-pinene and α-pinene. Peppermint oil is non-toxic and non-irritant in low dilutions, but sensitization may be a problem due to the menthol content. It can cause irritation to the skin and mucus membranes and should be kept well away from the eyes. Peppermint oil should be stored in closed containers kept in a dry place, avoiding sunshine and rain.

Composition	Method of Preparation	Caution
Oil of peppermint- 2 ml Precipitated calcium phosphate- 4 g Distilled water q.s.- 1000 ml	Triturate the oil of peppermint with the specified quantity of precipitated calcium phosphate, added the distilled water gradually, under constant trituration, and then filter.	It should be avoided during pregnancy and should not be used on children under seven.

Label

<table>
<tr><td colspan="3" align="center">PEPPERMINT WATER USP
(50 ml)</td></tr>
<tr>
<td>Composition:
Each 50 ml contains,
Oil of peppermint- 0.1 ml
Distilled water q.s.- 50 ml
Dose: 10 to 40 ml
Storage: Store in well-closed, light-resistant container in cool place to prevent the volatilization of peppermint oil.</td>
<td align="center">PEPMINT WATER
(Aromatic Water)
(Used as an antispasmodic and carminative in flatulence of the gastrointestinal tract, cramping and bloating, flatulent colic to relieve nausea and vomiting, and as a gentle aromatic stimulant)

PROTECT FROM SUN LIGHT
NOT FOR INJECTION</td>
<td>Mfg. Lic. No.- 5D/2010
Batch No.- BN 0115
Mfg. Date- Jun. 2011
Exp. Date- May. 2012
M.R.P.- Rs. 20.00
 (Inclusive of all taxes)
Mfd. By: YAVI PHARMA
KANPUR ROAD, LUCKNOW
UP- 226001</td>
</tr>
</table>

For the digestive system, peppermint oil is effective for a range of ailments, as it stimulates the gall bladder and the secretion of bile. It is used for colic, cramps, dyspepsia, spastic colon, flatulence and nausea and can relieve pain in cases of toothache, aching feet, rheumatism, neuralgia, muscular pains and painful periods. On the skin, peppermint oil is used to relieve skin irritation and itchiness and also helps to reduce skin redness, where inflammation is present. It is used for dermatitis, acne, ringworm, scabies, pruritus and also relieves itching, sunburn and inflammation of the skin, while at the same time having a cooling action. Peppermint oil is excellent for mental fatigue and depression, refreshing the spirit and stimulating mental agility and improving concentration. It is helpful in apathy, shock, headache, migraine, nervous stress, vertigo and faintness and in general respiratory disorders, as well as dry coughs, sinus congestion, asthma, bronchitis, pneumonia, tuberculosis and cholera.

5. Dill Water BPC

It is a preparation containing a volatile oil extracted from the dill plant, *Anethum graveolens* (Family- Umbelliferae). As the main constituents, dill contains at least 2.5% volatile oil (50% carvone, plus limonene, eugenol, anethole and others), flavonoids (including kaempferol), coumarins, xanthone derivatives, triterpenes, phenolic acids, protein and fixed oil. Dill is a common ingredient in gripe water, given to relieve wind and colic in babies. It is used to treat flatulence in infants and is helpful in stomach upsets, gas and bloating.

Composition	Method of Preparation
Oil of Dill- 12.5 ml Alcohol (90%)- 70 ml Distilled water q.s.- 100 ml	Dissolve the oil of dill in the alcohol then added the distilled water gradually, shake after each addition and then filtered. One part of this solution corresponds to about 40 parts of Dill Water.

Label

DILL WATER BPC (50 ml)		
Composition: Each 50 ml contains, Oil of Dill- 6.25 ml Ethanol (90%)- 35 ml Distilled water q.s.- 50 ml **Dose:** 1 to 10 ml **Storage:** Store in well-closed, light-resistant container in cool place to prevent the volatilization of dill oil.	**DILL WATER** (Aromatic Water) (Used as carminative, aromatic, stomachic, antispasmodic, galactagogue, in flatulent dyspepsia and specifically indicated for flatulent pain in infants) **PROTECT FROM SUN LIGHT** **NOT FOR INJECTION**	**Mfg. Lic. No.-** 5D/2010 **Batch No.-** GH 1025 **Mfg. Date-** Jun. 2011 **Exp. Date-** May. 2012 **M.R.P.-** Rs. 20.00 (Inclusive of all taxes) **Mfd. By:** YAVI PHARMA KANPUR ROAD, LUCKNOW UP- 226001

Marketed preparations

Active Ingredient(s)	Marketed Preparation (Manufacturer)
Rose Water	GULABARI **(DABAR)**
Dill Water	WOODWARD'S GRIPE WATER **(TTK HEALTH CARE LTD)**

EXERCISE - 1

Object

To prepare and submit 50 ml of Chloroform Water BP.

Theory

Aromatic waters are clear, saturated aqueous solutions of volatile oils or other aromatic or volatile substances. Aromatic waters may be prepared by distillation or solution of the aromatic substance, with or without the use of dispersing agents. Chloroform water is simple aromatic water, which contains purified water as a solvent but does not contain alcohol. It is saturated solution of chloroform in purified water.

Chloroform ($CHCl_3$) is a clear colorless liquid having specific gravity 1.474 to 1.479 and possesses characteristic odor with burning sweet taste. The solubility of chloroform is 1 in 800 parts of water. In the preparation of chloroform water, vigorous shaking is required to subdivide the chloroform in small globules for enhancing its solubility. Dispersing agents are not required in this preparation.

Formula

Ingredients	Quantity Required
Chloroform	2.5 ml
Purified water q.s. to	1000 ml

Apparatus

Glass beaker, measuring cylinder and volumetric pipette.

Procedure

Measure the required quantity of chloroform. Add sufficient quantity of purified water to make the required volume with constant stirring so that chloroform gets uniformly mixed. Transfer in clean amber colored glass container and close it tightly.

Category

Pharmaceutical aid.

Dose

15 to 30 ml.

Therapeutic Use

Chloroform water is used principally for perfuming, flavoring the formulation and also used as vehicle and preservative.

Storage

It should be stored in airtight, light resistance container in cool place. Aromatic waters deteriorate with time and it should be made in small quantities and protected from intense light and excessive heat.

Label

The label should have the caution 'PROTECT FROM SUN LIGHT' with red ink due to the presence of volatile constituents in the preparation; chloroform forms harmful phosgene gas in presence of light.

Specimen Label

The specimen label for Chloroform Water BP is given as:

<table>
<tr><td colspan="3" align="center">CHLOROFORM WATER BP
(50 ml)</td></tr>
<tr>
<td>Composition:
Each 50 ml contains,
Chloroform- 0.125 ml
Purified water q.s.- 50 ml
Dose: 15 to 30 ml
Storage: Store in airtight, light-resistant container in cool place.</td>
<td align="center">CHLORWATER
(Aromatic Water)
(Flavoring agent, vehicle and preservative)

PROTECT FROM SUN LIGHT
NOT FOR INJECTION</td>
<td>Mfg. Lic. No.- 2V/2010
Batch No.- YM 0512
Mfg. Date- Mar. 2011
Exp. Date- Feb. 2012
M.R.P.- Rs. 15.00
(Inclusive of all taxes)
Mfd. By: YAVI PHARMA
KANPUR ROAD, LUCKNOW
UP- 226001</td>
</tr>
</table>

EXERCISE - 2

Object

To prepare and submit 50 ml of Camphor Water BP.

Theory

Aromatic waters are saturated solutions of volatile oils (e.g. rose oil, peppermint oil) or other aromatic substances (e.g. camphor). Camphor $[C_{10}H_{16}O]$, is a ketone or a keto-tetrahydro-cymene, obtained from *Cinnamomum camphora*. Camphor occurs as a colorless, transparent, crystalline solid. It has a powerful penetrating odor, and pungent, somewhat bitter, taste, followed by a slight sensation of cold. It has specific gravity 0.986 to 0.996. Synthetic camphor differs from the natural camphor in being optically inactive instead of dextrorotatory. Camphor is readily soluble in alcohol (1 in 1.25), olive oil (1 in 4), and chloroform (4 in 1) but sparingly soluble in water (1 in 700). In the preparation of Camphor Water BP, alcohol acts as a distributing agent.

Formula

Ingredients	Quantity Required
Camphor	1 g
Ethanol (90%)	2 ml
Purified water q.s. to	1000 ml

Apparatus Used

Glass beaker, measuring cylinder and volumetric pipette.

Procedure

Measure the required quantity of camphor and dissolve in ethanol (90%). Add this solution in small quantities to the purified water with vigorous shaking after each addition. Afterward shake occasionally until all the camphor is dissolved. The addition of alcoholic solution to the purified water yields a finely divided precipitate of camphor, which redissolves easily on shaking. Transfer in clean amber colored glass container and close it tightly.

Category

Pharmaceutical aid.

Dose

30 to 60 ml.

Therapeutic Use

Camphor Water BP is used chiefly for flavoring purposes, but it has a mild carminative, diaphoretic, and expectorant action. Camphor Water BP is used as the vehicle in ophthalmic solutions owning to its ability to contribute refreshing, stimulating effect to the preparation.

Storage

Camphor Water BP should be stored in well-closed, light resistant container in cool place to prevent the volatilization of camphor.

Label

The label should have the caution 'PROTECT FROM SUN LIGHT' with red ink due to the presence of volatile constituents in the preparation.

Caution

Purified water should not be added to the alcoholic solution of camphor because this whole of the camphor will be precipitated out which will not redissolve easily on shaking. But the drop wise addition of alcoholic solution of camphor to the purified water will not cause this type of problem.

Specimen Label

The specimen label for Chloroform Water BP is given as:

<table>
<tr><td colspan="3" align="center">CAMPHOR WATER BP
(50 ml)</td></tr>
<tr>
<td valign="top">Composition:
Each 50 ml contains-
Camphor- 0.05 g
Ethanol (90%)- 0.1 ml
Purified water q.s.- 50 ml
Dose: 30 to 60 ml.
Storage: Store in airtight, light-resistant container in cool place.</td>
<td valign="top" align="center">CAMPWATER
(Aromatic Water)
(Flavouring agent, Mild carminative, Diaphoretic and Expectorant)

PROTECT FROM SUN LIGHT NOT FOR INJECTION</td>
<td valign="top">Mfg. Lic. No.- 5D/2010
Batch No.- CK 1523
Mfg. Date- Jun. 2011
Exp. Date- May. 2012
M.R.P.- Rs. 20.00
(Inclusive of all taxes)
Mfd. By: YAVI PHARMA KANPUR ROAD, LUCKNOW UP- 226001</td>
</tr>
</table>

EXERCISE - 3

Object

To prepare and submit 50 ml of Rose Water NF.

Theory

Aromatic waters are clear, saturated aqueous solutions of volatile substances. Rose Water NF is a saturated solution of the odoriferous active constituents of the flowers of *Rosa centifolia* (Family- Rosaceae) prepared by distilling the fresh flowers with water and separating the excess volatile oils from the clear water portion of the distillate. It is colorless, clear, strong, pleasant odor and taste of fresh rose blossoms, free from empyreuma, mustiness, or fungoid growths. It is neutral or slightly acidic in nature.

Formula

Ingredients	Quantity Required
Rose oil	2 ml
Ethanol (90%)	2 ml
Purified water q.s. to	100 ml

Apparatus Used

Glass beaker, measuring cylinder and volumetric pipette.

Procedure

Measure the required quantity of rose oil and dissolve in ethanol (90%). Add this solution in small quantities to the purified water with vigorous shaking after each addition. Afterward shake occasionally until all the rose oil is dissolved. Transfer in clean, transparent glass container and close it tightly.

Category

Pharmaceutical aid.

Dose

8 to 30 ml.

Therapeutic Use

Rose Water NF is used chiefly for flavoring purposes, but it has a mild carminative, diaphoretic, and expectorant action. Rose Water NF has an antioxidant activity. It cleanses tones and protects skin from harmful environmental impacts. It is capable of relieving skin ailments caused by circulation problems. It can reduce the redness and improve the general condition of the skin. It is suitable for all skin types. Rose Water NF is prescribed in lotions for its fragrant odor, and as a mild astringent. It is better known as an ingredient in cosmetics. It is also useful for hair. It makes hair glossy and healthy-looking.

Storage

Rose Water NF should be stored in well-closed, light resistant container in cool place to prevent the volatilization of rose oil.

Label

The label should have the caution 'PROTECT FROM SUN LIGHT' with red ink due to the presence of volatile constituents in the preparation.

Specimen Label

The specimen label for Rose Water NF is given as:

ROSE WATER NF (50 ml)		
Composition: Each 50 ml contains, Rose oil- 1 ml Ethanol (90 %)- 1 ml Purified water q.s.- 50 ml **Dose:** 8 to 30 ml. **Storage:** Store in airtight, light-resistant container in cool place.	**ROSE SHINE** (Aromatic Water) (Flavoring agent, Mild carminative, Diaphoretic and for skin ailments) **PROTECT FROM SUN LIGHT** **NOT FOR INJECTION**	**Mfg. Lic. No.-** 2J/2010 **Batch No.-** VD 0311 **Mfg. Date-** Aug. 2011 **Exp. Date-** July 2012 **M.R.P.-** Rs. 35.00 (Inclusive of all taxes) **Mfd. By:** YAVI PHARMA KANPUR ROAD, LUCKNOW UP- 226001

CHAPTER 2

SOLUTIONS

Solutions are liquid preparations that contain one or more chemical substances dissolved in a suitable solvent or mixture of mutually miscible solvents. A solution is a homogeneous mixture composed of two or more substances. In such a mixture, a solute is dissolved in another substance, known as a solvent. All solutions are characterized by interactions between the solvent phase and solute molecules or ions that result in a net decrease in free energy. The component present in large amount in a solution is termed as solvent and the component present in lesser amount is known as solute but irrespective of the relative amount of component, when a solid is dissolved in a liquid, the solid is treated as solute and liquid as solvent.

On the basis of their uses solutions may be categorized as oral, ophthalmic, otic or topical solutions. Solutions may also be categorized in other dosage form on the basis of their composition or use like **syrup** (aqueous solution of sugar), **elixir** (sweetened hydroalcoholic solution), **spirit** (alcoholic solution of aromatic substances), **aromatic water** (aqueous solution of aromatic substances) and **tincture** (alcoholic or hydroalcoholic extraction of crude drugs). Solutions have several advantages. Some of them are as follow:

1. Solutions being liquid are easier to swallow and are particularly acceptable for paediatric and geriatric use.
2. A drug must usually be in solution before it can be absorbed. If drug is administered in solution form, the therapeutic response will be faster than solid dosage form of drug.
3. A solution is a homogeneous system therefore the drug will be uniformly distributed throughout the preparation.
4. The drugs which can irritate and damage the gastric mucosa like aspirin and potassium chloride can be administered in solution form. Irritation is reduced by administration of a solution of drug due to its immediate dilution by gastric contents.

15

There are some disadvantages of solutions associated with the manufacture, transport, stability and administration of solution:

1. Solutions being liquid are bulky and are inconvenient to transport and store.

2. The stability of ingredients in aqueous solution is poorer than if formulated as solid dosage form.

3. Solutions are suitable media for microbial growth and therefore require the addition of a preservative.

4. When the taste of a drug is bitter and nauseating, a sweetening agent and flavoring agent is required to make the solution pleasant.

Solutions may be solid, liquid or gaseous but pharmaceutically important category is liquid solutions. The ability of one compound to dissolve in another compound is called solubility.

Solubility of an agent in a particular solvent indicates the maximum concentration to which a solution may be prepared with that agent and that solvent at a particular temperature. When a solute dissolves, the substance's intermolecular forces of attraction must be overcome by forces of attraction between the solute and solvent molecule.

Temperature is an important factor in determining the solubility of a drug and in preparing its solution. Most chemicals having positive heat of solution show increased solubility with an increase in temperature. The solubility of a pure chemical substance at a given temperature and pressure is constant however its rate of solution depends on the particle size of substance and the extent of agitation. General expressions of relative solubility as defined in IP (2007) are given in following table,

Descriptive Term	Parts of solvent required for 1 part of solute
Very soluble	Less than 1
Freely soluble	1-10
Soluble	10-30
Sparingly soluble	30-100
Slightly soluble	100-1000
Very slightly soluble	1000-10,000
Practically insoluble, or Insoluble	10,000 or more

Note: General expressions of relative solubility as defined in USP 30 (2007) are similar to that of IP (2007).

General Approaches for the Improvement of Aqueous Solubility

Although water is most common solvent yet some new therapeutic agents are not sufficiently soluble in it and hence approaches are utilized for the enhancement of solubility of drug in water.

A. Cosolvency

Cosolvency is a method of enhancing the solubility of a poorly soluble drug by addition of water miscible solvent in which the drug is very soluble. Such solvents are known as cosolvents. Commonly used cosolvents are ethanol, sorbitol, glycerin, propylene glycol and several polyethylene glycols (PEGs).

B. Solubilization

This term was introduced by Mc Bain in 1937. Solubilization has been defined as the spontaneous passage of poorly water soluble solute molecules in an aqueous solution of a soap in which a thermodynamically stable solution is formed. The mechanism for this phenomenon involves the property of surface active agent to form colloidal aggregates known as micelles. Solubilization occurs by virtue of the solute dissolving in or being adsorbed onto the micelles.

Thus the ability of surfactant solutions to dissolve or solubilize water insoluble drugs starts at the critical micelle concentration (CMC) and increases with the concentration of the micelles. When a surfactant with proper hydrophilic-lipophilic balance (HLB) values added to a liquid in very low concentrations, the solution behaves as an ideal one. Lyophilic surfactants with HLB values higher than 15 are considered to be the best solubilizing agents.

Solubilization concept has been employed pharmaceutically to solubilize water insoluble vitamins A, D and K as well as essential oils. Cholesterol can also be solubilized to an appreciable extent by the use of soaps. Some proprietary disinfectants like lysol (Cresol with Soap Solution), chloroxylenol solution and hexachlorophene liquid soap are formulated by the application of solubilization phenomenon.

C. pH modification

The solubility of chemotherapeutic agent (weak acid or weak base) can be markedly influenced by the pH of their environment. Through the application of the law of mass action, the solubility of weakly acid or basic drugs can be predicted, as a function of pH.

D. Complexation

Organic compounds in solution generally tend to associate with each other to some extent. Every substance has specific, reproducible equilibrium solubility in a given solvent at a given temperature. Any deviation from this inherent solubility must be due to the formation of a new species (complex) in solution. When complex formation occurs, the total solubility is equal to the inherent solubility of the uncomplexed drug plus the concentration of drug complex in solution.

E. Hydrotrophy

The term hydrotrophy denotes an increase in solubility of a drug in aqueous medium due to the presence of large amount of additives. Hydrotrophy is another type of solubilization in which the solute dissolves in oriented clusters of hydrotrophic agent. However, hydrotrophic solutions do not show colloidal properties. The possible mechanisms of hydrotrophy are considered to be solubilization, complexation and cosolvency, although the exact mechanism is not clearly understood.

Examples of this phenomenon include the increased solubility of adrenochrome monosemicarbazone with sodium salicylate, increased solubility of caffeine in presence of sodium benzoate, increased solubility of benzoic acid in presence of sodium benzoate and that of theophylline in presence of sodium acetate and sodium glycinate.

Except these examples, hydrotrophy dose not has much practical significance for pharmaceutical systems for enhancing the drug solubility probably due to the large amount (in the range of 20 to 50%) of additives necessary to produce modest increases in solubility.

F. Chemical Modification of the Drug

Many poorly soluble drugs can be chemically modified to their water soluble derivatives. Examples include the synthesis of the sodium phosphate salts of many corticosteroids like hydrocortisone, prednisolone and betamethasone. The solubility of betamethasone alcohol in water is 5.8 mg/100 ml at 25°C but the solubility of its disodium phosphate ester is found to be greater than 10 g/100 ml. Thus, over 1500 times enhancement in solubility of this drug can be achieved through chemical modification.

New modified drugs must be subjected to essentially the same testing protocol as the parent drug, including biological activity studies, acute and chronic toxicity, pharmaceutical evaluation, chemical purity and clinical testing. Hence this approach is justified only when no other method for enhancement of solubility is applicable.

Methods of Preparation

In pharmaceutical practice solutions are liquid preparations containing one or more chemical substances usually dissolved in water. Solutions are applied for specific therapeutic effect of solute either internally or externally. They vary in composition, method of preparation, potency, mode of administration, dose and therapeutic uses. The methods of preparation of solutions are as follow:

Simple Dissolution

Simple solutions are prepared by dissolving the solute in a suitable solvent with or without the application of heat e.g. calcium hydroxide solution, morphine hydrochloride solution.

Solution by Chemical Reaction

In this method the solutions are prepared by reaction of two or more solutes with each other in a suitable solvent e.g. aluminium subacetate solution.

Solution by Extraction

In this method, the active components of crude drugs are extracted with the help of suitable solvents. These preparations are known as extractive e.g. fluid extract and tinctures.

Therapeutic Uses

The therapeutic uses of different types of solutions depend on the drug/active ingredient present in that formulation e.g. aqueous Iodine Solution IP is a source of iodine so it can be useful in case of iodine deficiency disorders like goiter. Povidone-Iodine solution is used topically as a surgical scrub and non-irritating antiseptic solution. Another solution, Cresol with Soap Solution IP is used as a general disinfectant for hospital and domestic use.

Dose

The recommended dose of different types of solution depends on their respective potency and intended uses e.g. the recommended dose of Aqueous Iodine Solution IP (Lugol's solution) is 0.3-1 ml and that of Strong Ammonium Acetate Solution BP is 1 to 4 ml. A 1% solution of Cresol with Soap Solution IP may be applied to wash the wounds but 3-5% solution is used for sterilization of instruments.

Storage Conditions

The solutions should be stored in well-closed containers. In case of iodine preparations, the material of the container should be resistant to iodine.

Specific Labeling Requirement

Aqueous Iodine Oral Solution BP is dispensed in dilute form so the label should state that the solution should be well diluted before use. Alcoholic Iodine Solution BP is a cutaneous solution. So it should have the caution 'FOR EXTERNAL USE ONLY'. The label should also have the date after which the solution is not intended to be used.

Cresol with Soap Solution IP (Lysol) is a general disinfectant so the label should have the caution 'FOR EXTERNAL USE ONLY'. Cresol being a phenolic compound, light can affect the formulation so the label of Lysol solution should also have the caution 'PROTECT FROM LIGHT'. Being a topical antiseptic solution, the label of Povidone-Iodine Solution BP should have the caution 'FOR EXTERNAL USE ONLY'.

Examples of Solutions

1. Aqueous Iodine Oral Solution BP

It is an extemporaneous preparation. Iodine content of this solution varies from 4.75-5.25% w/v and that of potassium iodide content 9.5-10.5% w/v.

Composition	Method of Preparation
Iodine - 50 g Potassium Iodide - 100 g Purified water (freshly boiled and cooled) q.s.- 1000 ml	This solution can be prepared by dissolving Iodine and Potassium Iodide in freshly boiled and cooled purified water sufficient to produce 1000 ml.

Label

<table>
<tr><td colspan="3" align="center">AQUEOUS IODINE ORAL SOLUTION BP
(50 ml)</td></tr>
<tr>
<td>Composition:
Each 50 ml contains,
Iodine- 2.5 g
Potassium Iodide - 5 g
Purified water q.s.- 50 ml
Dose: 15 ml (well diluted before use)
Storage: Store in airtight, light-resistant container in cool place to prevent the volatilization of iodine.</td>
<td align="center">AQUA IODINE
(Solution)
(Used as a source of iodine in the treatment of goiter)

PROTECT FROM SUN LIGHT
NOT FOR INJECTION</td>
<td>Mfg. Lic. No.- 2P/2010
Batch No.- CD 0502
Mfg. Date- July, 2011
Exp. Date- June 2012
M.R.P.- Rs. 20.00
(Inclusive of all taxes)
Mfd. By: YAVI PHARMA
KANPUR ROAD, LUCKNOW
UP- 226001</td>
</tr>
</table>

2. Aqueous Iodine Solution (Lugol's Solution) IP

Iodine is very slightly soluble in water but it is soluble in water in presence of potassium iodide due to the formation of polyiodides complex. These polyiodides improve the solubility of iodine and produce a stable aqueous iodine solution. Aqucous Iodine Solution IP contains 5% w/v of iodine and 10% w/v of potassium iodide.

Composition	Method of Preparation	Caution
Iodine - 5 g Potassium Iodide - 10 g Purified water q.s.- 100 ml	Weigh the required quantity of iodine and potassium iodide separately. Triturate the iodine into fine powder in a glass mortar. Dissolve separately potassium iodide in a small portion of water. To this solution, add iodine and dissolve by continuous stirring with glass rod. When iodine dissolve completely, add sufficient quantity of purified water to produce 100 ml of solution.	Metallic containers should not be used for the storage of the preparation because iodine being an oxidizing agent, it oxidizes iron and converts into ferrous iodide. Metallic spatula should not be used for handling of iodine.

Label

AQUEOUS IODINE SOLUTION IP		
(50 ml)		
Composition: Each 50 ml contains, Iodine- 2.5 g Potassium Iodide - 5 g Purified water q.s.- 50 ml **Dose:** 15 ml at night **Storage:** Store in well-closed iodine resistant containers.	**AQUADINE** (Solution) (Internally, used as a source of iodine in the treatment of goiter and externally, used as antiseptic) **PROTECT FROM SUN LIGHT** **NOT FOR INJECTION**	**Mfg. Lic. No.-** 2Q/2010 **Batch No.-** CM 0510 **Mfg. Date-** Aug., 2011 **Exp. Date-** July 2012 **M.R.P.-** Rs. 25.00 (Inclusive of all taxes) **Mfd. By:** YAVI PHARMA KANPUR ROAD, LUCKNOW UP- 226001

3. Alcoholic Iodine Solution BP

Alcoholic Iodine Solution BP is an extemporaneous preparation. It has iodine content 2.4-2.7% w/v, potassium iodide content 2.4-2.7% w/v and ethanol content 83-88% v/v. When iodine tincture is prescribed, Alcoholic Iodine Solution BP shall be dispensed.

Composition	Method of Preparation	Caution
Iodine - 25 g Potassium Iodide - 25 g Purified water- 25 ml Ethanol (90%) q.s.- 100 ml	Dissolve potassium iodide in purified water. To this solution, add iodine and dissolve by continuous stirring with glass rod. When iodine dissolve completely, add sufficient quantity of alcohol to produce 100 ml of solution.	Metallic containers should not be used for the storage of the preparation. Metallic spatula should not be used for handling of iodine.

Label

ALCOHOLIC IODINE SOLUTION BP **(50 ml)**		
Composition: Each 50 ml contains, Iodine - 12.5 g Potassium Iodide - 12.5 g Purified water - 12.5 ml Ethanol (90%) q.s.- 50 ml **Dose:** 15 ml **Storage:** Store in well-closed iodine resistant containers.	**ALCODINE** (Solution) (Used as antiseptic) **PROTECT FROM SUN LIGHT** **NOT FOR INJECTION**	**Mfg. Lic. No.-** 5M/2010 **Batch No.-** KJ 0110 **Mfg. Date-** Mar., 2011 **Exp. Date-** Feb. 2012 **M.R.P.-** Rs. 22.00 (Inclusive of all taxes) **Mfd. By:** YAVI PHARMA KANPUR ROAD, LUCKNOW UP- 226001

4. Povidone-Iodine Solution BP

It is a cutaneous solution having the deep brown color and characteristic odor of iodine. The content of available iodine in Povidone-Iodine Solution BP varies from 0.85-1.2% w/v.

Composition	Method of Preparation
Iodinated Povidone- 5 g Purified water-100 ml	It is prepared either by dissolving Iodinated Povidone in purified water or by the interaction between Iodine and Povidone (polyvinylpyrrolidone).

<table>
<tr><td colspan="3" align="center">Label</td></tr>
</table>

POVIDONE-IODINE SOLUTION BP		
(50 ml)		
Composition:	**PODINE**	**Mfg. Lic. No.-** 7D/2010
Each 50 ml contains,	(Solution)	**Batch No.-** VN 0178
Iodinated Povidone - 2.5 g	(Used as antiseptic)	**Mfg. Date-** Mar. 2011
Purified water q.s.- 50 ml		**Exp. Date-** Feb. 2012
Dose: As directed by physician		**M.R.P.-** Rs. 28.00
Storage: Store in well-closed	**PROTECT FROM SUN LIGHT**	(Inclusive of all taxes)
iodine resistant containers.	**NOT FOR INJECTION**	**Mfd. By:** YAVI PHARMA KANPUR ROAD, LUCKNOW UP- 226001

5. Cresol with Soap Solution (Lysol Solution) IP

Cresol with Soap Solution IP is an amber-colored to reddish-brown liquid. It has the odor of cresol and soapy to touch. Cresol with soap solution contains not less than 47% v/v and not more than 53% v/v of cresol. Cresol is a mixture of its 3 isomers (ortho, meta and para cresol).

Composition	Method of Preparation	Caution
Cresol- 50 ml Vegetable oil- 18 ml Potassium hydroxide- 4 g Purified water q.s.- 100 ml	It is prepared by the saponification of a mixture of cresol with vegetable oils such as cotton seed, linseed, soyabean or similar oils but excluding coconut and palm karnel oils. Alternatively, the mixed fatty acids derived from these oils may be used.	Since cresol is a phenolic compound and caustic in nature so it should be handled carefully.

<table>
<tr><td colspan="3" align="center">Label</td></tr>
<tr><td colspan="3" align="center">CRESOL WITH SOAP SOLUTION IP
(50 ml)</td></tr>
<tr>
<td>Composition:
Each 50 ml contains,
Cresol- 25 ml
Purified water q.s.- 50 ml
Dose: 0.2% solution as vaginal douche, 1% solution for wounds wash and 3-5% solution for sterilization of instruments.
Storage: Store in a well-closed container and protected from light.</td>
<td align="center">YAVISOL
(Solution)
(Used as antiseptic and general disinfectant for hospital and domestic use)

PROTECT FROM SUN LIGHT
FOR EXTERNAL USE ONLY</td>
<td>Mfg. Lic. No.- 9E/2010
Batch No.- KK 0620
Mfg. Date- May, 2011
Exp. Date- Apr. 2012
M.R.P.- Rs. 30.00
(Inclusive of all taxes)
Mfd. By: YAVI PHARMA KANPUR ROAD, LUCKNOW UP- 226001</td>
</tr>
</table>

6. Calcium Hydroxide Topical Solution USP

It contains in each 100 ml, not less than 140 mg of calcium hydroxide. The solubility of calcium hydroxide varies with the temperature at which the solution is stored, so in the preparation of Calcium Hydroxide Topical Solution USP cool purified water is used as a solvent because calcium hydroxide is less soluble in hot water than in cold water. Its solubility is about 170 mg per 100 ml at 15°C and lesser at higher temperature. The official concentration is based upon the temperature of 25°C. This solution absorbs carbon dioxide from the air and forms a film of calcium carbonate on the surface of the solution. When heated, solution becomes turbid due to the separation of calcium hydroxide and clear again on cooling.

Composition	Method of Preparation	Caution
Calcium hydroxide - 3 g Purified water (cool) q.s.- 1000 ml	Add the required quantity of calcium hydroxide to 1000 ml of cool purified water and agitate the mixture vigorously and repeatedly during 1 hour. Allow the excess calcium hydroxide to settle. Use only the clear supernatant.	The undissolved portion is not suitable for preparing additional quantities of Calcium Hydroxide Topical Solution USP.

Label

<table>
<tr><td colspan="3" align="center">CALCIUM HYDROXIDE TOPICAL SOLUTION USP
(50 ml)</td></tr>
<tr>
<td>Composition:
Each 50 ml contains,
Calcium hydroxide – 0.15 g
Purified water q.s.- 50 ml
Storage: Store in well-filled, tight containers, at a temperature not exceeding 25°C.</td>
<td align="center">CALTOP
(Topical Solution)

PROTECT FROM SUN LIGHT
NOT FOR INJECTION</td>
<td>Mfg. Lic. No.- 1D/2010
Batch No.- LN 0110
Mfg. Date- Sept. 2011
Exp. Date- Aug. 2012
M.R.P.- Rs. 19.00
(Inclusive of all taxes)
Mfd. By: YAVI PHARMA KANPUR ROAD, LUCKNOW UP- 226001</td>
</tr>
</table>

7. Strong Ammonium Acetate Solution BP

Strong Ammonium Acetate Solution BP is an extemporaneous preparation and has ammonium acetate content about 55-60% w/v. Its relative density is 1.085 to 1.095.

Composition	Method of Preparation
Glacial acetic acid- 453 g Ammonium bicarbonate- 470 g Strong ammonia solution- 100 ml Purified water (freshly boiled and cooled) q.s.- 1000 ml	Dissolve the ammonium bicarbonate by adding gradually to the glacial acetic acid previously diluted with 350 ml of purified water. Add strong ammonia solution until 0.05 ml of the resulting solution diluted with 0.5 ml of water gives a full blue color with 0.05 ml of bromothymol blue solution and a full yellow color with 0.05 ml of thymol blue solution. Add sufficient purified water to produce 1000 ml. **Note-** Indicators, bromothymol blue and thymol blue are used to adjust the pH 7.6 to 8.1.

Label

<table>
<tr><td colspan="3" align="center">STRONG AMMONIUM ACETATE SOLUTION BP
(50 ml)</td></tr>
<tr>
<td>Composition:
Each 50 ml contains,
Glacial acetic acid- 453 g
Ammonium bicarbonate- 470 g
Strong ammonia solution- 100 ml
Purified water q.s.-1000 ml
Dose: 1 to 4 ml
Storage: Store in a well-closed lead-free glass container in cool place.</td>
<td align="center">AMCETATE
(Solution)
(Used as diaphoretic)

PROTECT FROM SUN LIGHT

NOT FOR INJECTION</td>
<td>Mfg. Lic. No.- 5M/2010
Batch No.- KJ 0110
Mfg. Date- Mar. 2011
Exp. Date- Feb. 2012
M.R.P.- Rs. 22.00
(Inclusive of all taxes)
Mfd. By: YAVI PHARMA KANPUR ROAD, LUCKNOW UP- 226001</td>
</tr>
</table>

Marketed Preparations

Active Ingredient(s)	Marketed Preparation (Manufacturer)
Sodium chloride	**BASOL** (CADILA), **KORED DPS** (DEY'S)
Lactulose	**LOOZ** (INTAS), **OSMOWIN** (WIN MEDICARE), **RAPIDUCE** (FDC)
Clotrimazole	**CANESTEN** (BAYER), **SURFAZ** (FRANCO-INDIAN)
Tolnaftate	**TOLSOL** (JAGSONPAL)
Cetrimide	**CETRIMIDE** (NICHOLAS), **GERMISOL** (AGRAWAL PHARMA)
Minoxidil	**MINTOP** (DR.REDD'S LAB), **MANDIL** (ZEE LAB), **GROMANE** (ALIDAC), **HAIREX** (KOPRAN), **MORR** (INTAS)
Ketoconazole	**KETOSA** (SARMAIN), **KONAZ** (TALENT INDIA), **NIZRAL** (JOHNSON & JOHNSON), **NUKET** (LANCER PHARMA)
Povidone-iodine	**BETADINE** (WIN MEDICARE), **WOKADINE** (WOCKHARDT), **ALPHADINE** (NICHOLAS), **POVID SOLUTION** (BLISS), **BIPDINE** (BIONET INDIA)
Povidone-iodine and metronidazole	**POVIMET** (DRAKT PHARMA), **REDRESS** (RBS PHARMA)
Iodine	**IOPREP** (JOHNSON & JOHNSON)
Erythromycin	**AKNEMYCIN PLUS** (BOOTS PIRAMAL)
Chlorhexidine	**SAVLON** (JOHNSON & JOHNSON)
Podophyllotoxin	**CONDYLINE** (ELDER)
Sulphacetamide	**ALBUCID** (ALLERGAN), **ANDRIMIDE** (INTAS), **OPACID** (DEY'S), **SCARMIDE** (OSCAR REMEDIES), **ZINCOREN** (INDOCO)
Ofloxacin	**BESTOFLOX-D** (BESTOCHEM), **ENTOF** (DEY'S), **EXOCIN** (ALLERGAN), **OFLOTAS** (INTAS)
Ciprofloxacin	**ADIFLOX** (INTAS), **ALCIPRO** (ALKEM), **CIPLOX-D** (CIPLA), **CEPROLEN** (INDOCO), **CIPZY** (ZEE LAB)

EXERCISE - 4

Object

To prepare and submit 50 ml Cresol with Soap Solution (Lysol Solution) IP.

Theory

Cresol is a mixture of its three isomers (ortho, meta and para-cresol). The solubility of cresol is about 3% v/v but this preparation contains 50% v/v cresol so for dissolving this high proportion of cresol, some solubilizing agent is required. In this preparation solubilizing agent, soap is formed by the interaction of vegetable oil having fatty acids with potassium hydroxide (saponification). Vegetable oils such as cotton seed, linseed, soyabean or similar oils can be used, excluding coconut and palm karnel oils. Alternatively, the mixed fatty acids derived from these oils may be used. The cresol is mixed only after the completion of the reaction between vegetable oil and potassium hydroxide.

Saponification process can be hastened if part of the vegetable oil is replaced by oleic acid, which reacts with alkali quickly. The preparation can be further simplified by replacing the oil and alkali by soft soap. Cresol with Soap Solution IP (Lysol Solution) is an amber-colored to reddish-brown liquid. It has the odor of cresol and soapy to touch and it contains not less than 47% v/v and not more than 53% v/v of cresol.

Formula

Ingredients	Quantity Required
Cresol	50 ml
Vegetable oil	18 g
Potassium hydroxide	4.2 g
Purified water q.s. to	100 ml

Apparatus

Glass beaker, conical flask, measuring cylinder and volumetric pipette.

Procedure

Measure the required quantity of cresol and dissolve in 50% of purified water. Add required quantity of vegetable oil to this solution and heat on a water bath and mix thoroughly. Continue reflux heating until a small portion dissolves in water without separation of oily drops (i.e. the formation of soap is completed). Add cresol and mixed thoroughly. Then add sufficient purified water to produce the required volume of the preparation. Transfer it in clean amber colored glass container and close it tightly.

Category

Disinfectant.

Dose

A 0.2% Lysol Solution IP may be used as vaginal douche. A 1% solution of it may be applied to wash the wounds and 3-5% of its solution is used for sterilization of instruments.

Therapeutic Use

Cresol with Soap Solution IP is used as a general disinfectant for hospital and domestic use.

Storage

It should be stored in well-closed, light resistant narrow mouthed bottle in cool place.

Label

Cresol with Soap Solution IP is a general disinfectant so the label should have the caution 'FOR EXTERNAL USE ONLY'. Since cresol is a phenolic compound, light can affect the formulation so the label should also have the direction 'PROTECT FROM LIGHT' with red ink.

Caution

Since cresol is a phenolic compound and caustic in nature so it should be handled carefully.

Specimen Label

The specimen label for Cresol with Soap Solution IP is given as:

<table>
<tr><td colspan="3" align="center">CRESOL WITH SOAP SOLUTION (LYSOL SOLUTION) IP
(50 ml)</td></tr>
<tr>
<td>Composition:
Each 50 ml contains,
Cresol- 25 ml
Purified water q.s.- 50 ml
Storage: Store in well-closed, light resistant narrow mouthed bottle in cool place.</td>
<td align="center">YAVISOL
(Solution)
Disinfectant
(General disinfectant for hospital and domestic use)
PROTECT FROM SUN LIGHT
FOR EXTERNAL USE ONLY</td>
<td>Mfg. Lic. No.- 5K/2010
Batch No.- UM 0311
Mfg. Date- Feb. 2011
Exp. Date- Mar. 2012
M.R.P.- Rs. 30.00
(Inclusive of all taxes)
Mfd. By: YAVI PHARMA
KANPUR ROAD, LUCKNOW UP- 226001</td>
</tr>
</table>

EXERCISE - 5

Object

To prepare and submit 50 ml Strong Ammonium Acetate Solution BP.

Theory

Strong Ammonium Acetate Solution BP is an extemporaneous preparation. Content of ammonium acetate in Strong Ammonium Acetate Solution BP is about 55-60% w/v. Its relative density is 1.085 to 1.095 and pH of a 10% v/v solution is 7-8. When ammonium acetate solution or dilute ammonium acetate solution is prescribed, Strong Ammonium Acetate Solution BP diluted to 8 times its volume with freshly boiled and cooled purified water, shall be dispensed.

Formula

Ingredients	Quantity Required
Ammonium bicarbonate	470 g
Glacial acetic acid	453 g
Strong ammonia solution	100 ml or sufficient quantity
Purified water (freshly boiled and cooled) q.s. to	1000 ml

Apparatus

Glass beaker, measuring cylinder and volumetric pipette.

Procedure

Dissolve the required quantity of ammonium bicarbonate by adding gradually to the glacial acetic acid, previously diluted with 350 ml of purified water. Add sufficient quantity of strong ammonia solution until 0.05 ml of the resulting solution diluted with 0.5 ml of water gives a full blue color with 0.05 ml of bromothymol blue solution and a full yellow color with 0.05 ml of thymol blue solution. Add sufficient purified water to produce 1000 ml of the preparation.

Note: The preparation is made alkaline with pII range 7.6 to 8.1. The pH is adjusted by using two indicators like bromothymol blue and thymol blue.

Category

Diaphoretic.

Dose

1 to 4 ml.

Therapeutic Use

Strong Ammonium Acetate Solution BP is used as diaphoretic.

Storage

Strong Ammonium Acetate Solution BP should be kept in well-closed lead-free glass containers in cool place to prevent the loss of volatile constituents.

Label

The label should state the date after which the solution is not intended to be used and the conditions under which it should be stored. The label should have the caution 'PROTECT FROM SUN LIGHT' in red ink due to the presence of volatile constituents in the preparation.

Specimen Label

The specimen label for Strong Ammonium Acetate Solution BP is given as:

<table>
<tr><td colspan="3" align="center">STRONG AMMONIUM ACETATE SOLUTION BP
(50 ml)</td></tr>
<tr>
<td valign="top">
Composition:
Each 50 ml contains,
Ammonium bicarbonate- 23.5 g
Glacial acetic acid- 22.65 g
Strong ammonia solution- 5 ml
Purified water q.s.- 50 ml
Dose: 1 to 4 ml
Storage: Store in well-closed lead-free glass container in cool place.
</td>
<td valign="top" align="center">
AMMACETA
(Solution)
Diaphoretic

PROTECT FROM SUN LIGHT
NOT FOR INJECTION
</td>
<td valign="top">
Mfg. Lic. No.- 4C/2010
Batch No.- NG 0741
Mfg. Date- Oct. 2011
Exp. Date- Sep. 2012
M.R.P.- Rs. 23.00
(Inclusive of all taxes)
Mfd. By: YAVI PHARMA
KANPUR ROAD, LUCKNOW UP- 226001
</td>
</tr>
</table>

CHAPTER 3

SYRUPS

Syrups are concentrated aqueous preparations of a sugar or sugar substitute with or without flavoring agents and medicinal substances. Syrup is essentially sugar dissolved in water, with or without flavors.

A syrup is a thick, viscous liquid containing a large amount of dissolved sugars, but showing little tendency to deposit crystals. The viscosity arises from the multiple hydrogen bonds, between the dissolved sugar, which has many hydroxyl groups and the water.

Syrups containing flavoring agents but no medicinal substances are called **nonmedicated** or **flavored syrups** e.g. Cherry Syrup, Orange Syrup, Raspberry Syrup, Cocoa Syrup etc. These syrups are intended to serve as pleasant tasting vehicles for medicinal substances to be added in the extemporaneous compounding of prescriptions. Flavored syrups are made by adding flavoring matter to simple syrup. For instance, *Syrupus aromaticus* is prepared by adding certain quantities of orange flavor and cinnamon water to simple syrup.

Syrups containing a therapeutic agent are known as **medicated syrups**. Medicated syrups are commercially prepared by combining each of the individual components of the syrup such as sucrose, purified water, flavoring agents, coloring agents, the therapeutic agent (medicinal substance) and other necessary and desirable ingredients. Naturally medicated syrups are employed in therapeutics for the value of medicinal agent present in the syrup.

Syrups provide a pleasant means of administering a liquid form of a disagreeable tasting drug. They are particularly affective in the administration of drugs to youngsters, since their pleasant taste usually dissipates any reluctance on the part of the child to take the medicine. The syrups contain little or no alcohol which adds to their favour among parents.

Any water soluble drug that is stable in aqueous solution may be added to a flavored syrup. During the formulation the compatibility issues between drug and other formulative component of the syrup must be considered. Certain flavored syrups have an acidic medium so proper selection must be made to ensure the stability of any added medicinal agent. Medications most frequently administered as medicated syrups are antitussive agents and antihistamines.

Glucose syrup is the concentrated solution of sugars from the acid or enzymatic hydrolysis of starch (usually maize or potato starch); a mixture of varying amounts of glucose, maltose, and glucose complexes. Usually 70% total solids by weight, containing glucose, maltose and oligomers of glucose of 3, 4 or more units.

The saccharometer, a weighted glass bulb that floats upright in the syrup so that a figure can be read off a scale, has been used since the early nineteenth century for measuring syrup density (its sugar content).

Syrup Components

Most of the syrups have the following components along with purified water and medicinal substance, if any:

(a) Sugar or Sugar Substitutes (Artificial Sweeteners)

Traditionally syrups are composed of sucrose (usually between 60% and 80%) and purified water. Due to the inherent sweetness and moderately high viscosity of these systems, the addition of other sweetening agents and viscosity-modifying agents is not required. Although most frequently used sugar in syrups is sucrose, it may be replaced in whole or in part by other sugars like dextrose or non-sugars like sorbitol, glycerine and propylene glycol. Some non glycogenetic substances like methylcellulose and hydroxyethylcellulose can also be used in place of glycogenic substances for medications used by diabetic patients. Syrups contain a high proportion of sucrose to attain not only desirable sweetness and viscosity but also for inherent stability (physical as well as microbial). Sucrose of pharmaceutical grade is always preferred.

The concentration of sucrose in sugar based syrups is very important. Syrup IP is 66.7% w/w sucrose solution while Syrup USP is 85% w/v (corresponding to 64.74% w/w) solution of sucrose in purified water.

Syrups can contain lower concentrations of sugars but will often include sufficient of a polyhydric alcohol such as sorbitol, glycerol or propylene glycol in order to maintain a high osmotic gradient. In addition, by acting as cosolvents they will help to prevent crystallization and to maintain solubility of all ingredients.

(b) Preservatives

In addition, the high concentration of sucrose and associated unavailability of water ensure that the addition of preservatives is not required. As the concentration of sucrose is reduced from the upper limit through dilution, the addition of preservatives may be required. A dilute solution of sucrose supports microbial growth but if syrup contains about 65% w/w or more of sugar, it will retard the growth of microorganisms. Conversely, in sugar-free syrups, (syrups in which sucrose have been substituted at least in part by polyhydric alcohol) and in traditional syrups (syrups which contain lower concentrations of sucrose), the addition of preservatives is required.

Typical examples of commonly used preservatives include, mixtures of parahydroxybenzoate esters (usually methylhydroxybenzoate and propylhydroxybenzoate in a ratio of 9:1). The typical concentration range of preservatives is 0.1-0.2% w/v. It is important to note that the preservative efficacy of these preservatives may be decreased in the presence of hydrophilic polymers (generally employed to enhance viscosity), due to an interaction of the preservative with the polymer. This effect is negated by increasing the overall preservative concentration. Other preservatives that are employed include benzoic acid (0.1-0.2%) or sodium benzoate (0.1-0.2%).

(c) Flavoring Agents

Syrups can be flavored with the help of synthetic flavorant or with natural materials like volatile oils, vanillin etc. to impart pleasant taste to them. These are employed whenever the unpalatable taste of a therapeutic agent is apparent, even in the presence of the sweetening agents. The flavors may be of natural origin (e.g. peppermint, lemon, herbs and spices) and are available as oils, extracts, spirits or aqueous solutions. Alternatively, a wide range of synthetic flavors are available that offer advantages over their natural counterparts in terms of purity, availability, stability and solubility. The concentration of flavor in oral syrups is that which provides the required degree of taste-masking.

(d) Coloring Agents

Colors are generally natural or synthetic water soluble, photo-stable ingredients. To enhance the aesthetic value of syrup, a coloring agent is used. The colorant used should be generally water soluble, non-reactive with other components of the syrup and should be stable at the pH range and under intense light. These are selected according to the flavor of the preparation. For example, mint-flavored formulations are commonly a green color, whereas in banana-flavored solutions a yellow color is commonly employed. Such ingredients must not chemically or physically interact with the other components of the formulation.

Methods of Preparation

On the basis of physical and chemical characteristics of the ingredients, the syrups can be prepared by one of the following methods-

1. Hot Process (Solution with the Aid of Heat)

This method is used when the active component is heat stable (non-volatile) and it is desired to prepare the syrup as quickly as possible. In this method, the sucrose is added to purified water and heated on water bath until the sugar is dissolved. Then other heat stable components are added to hot syrup, the mixture is allowed to cool and its final volume is adjusted to desired weight or volume by addition of purified water. The use of heat facilitates rapid solution of sugar but excessive heating leads to the inversion of sucrose and hydrolyzed into monosaccharide dextrose (glucose) and fructose (levulose). The colorless syrup darkens due to the effect of heat on the levulose portion of invert sugar.

Due to possibility of decomposition by heat, syrups can not be sterilized by autoclaving. The use of boiled purified water during the preparation of syrup can enhance its permanency. The Simple Syrup BP is prepared by adding 1 kg of refined sugar to 500 ml of boiling distilled water, heating until it is dissolved and subsequently adding boiling distilled water until the total weight is 1.5 kg. The specific gravity of the syrup should be 1.33. This is a 66° Brix solution. Simple Syrup IP, Acacia Syrup NF, Cocoa Syrup NF and Tolu Syrup IP are prepared by this method.

2. Cold Process (Solution by Agitation without The Aid of Heat)

This method is applicable for preparing the syrup containing heat sensitive ingredients. On small scale, sucrose and other formulative ingredients are dissolved in purified water by placing the ingredients in a vessel having larger capacity than the volume of the syrup to be prepared and thorough agitation of the mixture.

This method is more time consuming but the product has maximum stability. For large scale production mechanical stirrers or agitators are used. It is a best way to add solid ingredients into syrup that they should be dissolved in a minimal amount of purified water and incorporate the resulting solution into the syrup. Ferrous Sulphate Syrup USP is prepared by this method.

3. Percolation

In this method sucrose is placed in a suitable percolator and purified water is allowed to pass slowly through the sucrose. The rate of percolation regulates the rate of dissolution of sucrose. The neck of the percolator is packed with cotton. To get the complete dissolution of sucrose, the percolate may be returned back to the percolator. Cotton plug and inside of the percolator should be rinsed with purified water. Final volume is adjusted by adding more purified water. Syrup USP and Ipecac Syrup are prepared by this method.

4. Addition of Sucrose to a Medicated Liquid or to a Flavored Liquid

In this method sucrose is added to a medicated liquid like tincture or fluid extract to prepare the syrup. If the tincture or fluid extract is miscible with the aqueous preparation, it may be added directly to simple syrup or flavored syrup.

The tincture or fluid extract (alcoholic or hydroalcoholic preparation) contains alcohol soluble constituents. Addition of syrup in tincture or fluid extract may cause precipitation of alcohol soluble constituents due to the dilution with water.

Advantages of Syrups

1. Syrup retards oxidation. It is partially hydrolyzed into reducing sugars, which act as antioxidant and prevent the oxidation of drug.
2. Syrup prevents the growth of microorganisms due to high osmotic pressure.
3. Syrup is used as a sweetening agent for masking the bitter, saline and nauseous taste of the drugs.
4. Syrups are better acceptable by paediatric patient.
5. Syrups are also used as vehicle in various pharmaceutical preparations.

Disadvantages of Syrups

1. In case of diluted syrups or syrups containing less than 66.7% w/w, it leads to microbial growth hence it requires addition of extra preservatives.
2. If syrups are highly concentrated, it leads to crystallization of sucrose.

Therapeutic Uses

Syrups are palatable and due to the sweetness of sugar it is a valuable vehicle for the administration of nauseous and bitter substances. Syrup has high osmotic pressure that prevents the growth of microorganisms and serves as a preservative. Syrup retards oxidation as it is partly hydrolyzed into reducing sugar like levulose and dextrose, which act as antioxidants. Syrups are used as base for various flavored and medicated syrups. For example, Tolu Syrup is used as a cough expectorant and Orange Syrup as a flavoring agent. Syrups can also be used in the manufacturing of other preparations like elixirs or mixtures. Codeine Phosphate Syrup IP is used as analgesic and antitussive. Chlorpheniramine Maleate Syrup is used as antihistaminic. Piperazine Citrate Syrup USP is used as an anthelmintic in the treatment of pin worms and round worms. Compound Ferrous Phosphate Syrup BPC (Parrish's Syrup) is used as a haematinic tonic.

Syrups can also be used as viscosity-enhancing agents due to their inherent viscosity. They can also be used as a sweetening agent in sugar confectionery. They add a sweet flavor. The chemical and physical properties of syrups make them exceptionally useful in industrial baking. Nutritionally, simple syrups provide concentrated energy.

Dose

The recommended dose of different syrups depends on the medicament/active constituents they contain e.g. the doses of Codeine Phosphate Syrup IP, Chlorpheniramine Maleate Syrup and Compound Ferrous Phosphate Syrup BPC are 2.5-10 ml, 4-6 ml and 2-8 ml respectively.

Storage conditions

Syrups should be stored at a temperature not exceeding 25°C. All official syrups should be stored in well-dried, completely filled and carefully stoppered bottles in a cool and dark place. Syrups which are concentrated but not supersaturated are self-preserving as they are capable of resisting bacterial growth by virtue of their osmotic effect.

When the concentration of sucrose in syrup is low then preservatives like benzoic acid, sodium benzoate and methylparaben are used in proper concentration. Use of sterilized containers and closures is an effective way to check the growth of microorganisms in the syrup.

A problem with the storage and use of syrups involves the crystallization of the sugar within the screw cap used to seal the containers, thereby preventing its release. It can be avoided by the addition of polyhydric alcohols or by the inclusion of invert sugar.

Specific labeling requirement

The label should have the direction 'SHAKE WELL BEFORE USE' and 'PROTECT FROM SUN LIGHT AND HEAT' in red ink.

Contraindication

Syrups having sugar should not be given to the diabetic patients. Such patients should be given syrups containing the non-sugars like methylcellulose and hydroxyethylcellulose. Syrup preserved with hydroxybenzoate (parabens) esters may be incompatible with methadone hydrochloride.

Examples of Syrups

1. Invert Syrup BP

Invert Syrup BP has a mixture of glucose and fructose. It is a clear, colorless to pale straw-colored syrupy liquid. It is odorless or almost odorless and has a sweet taste. It is miscible with water, producing a clear solution; it dissolves in ethanol (96%) with the formation of an insoluble residue. The degree of inversion is at least 95%. The content of reducing sugars, expressed as invert sugar should not be less than 67% w/w. Its solution in water is laevorotatory and has a pH 5.0 to 6.0. Refractive index of Invert Syrup BP is 1.4608 to 1.4630 and weight per ml is 1.338 to 1.344 g.

Composition	Method of Preparation
Sucrose- 66.7 g Mineral acid- q.s. Calcium carbonate or Sodium carbonate- q.s. Purified water q.s.- 100 ml	It is prepared by hydrolyzing a 66.7% w/w solution of sucrose with a suitable mineral acid, such as hydrochloric acid, and neutralizing the resulting solution using calcium carbonate or sodium carbonate.

Label

INVERT SYRUP BP (50 ml)		
Composition: Each 50 ml contains, Sucrose- 33.35 g Purified water q.s.- 50 ml **Dose:** 15 ml **Storage:** Store in airtight, light-resistant container at a temperature of 35°C-45°C.	**INVESYR** (Syrup) (Used as sweetening agent) **PROTECT FROM SUN LIGHT AND HEAT** **SHAKE WELL BEFORE USE**	**Mfg. Lic. No.-** 4K/2010 **Batch No.-** CV 0144 **Mfg. Date-** Jan. 2011 **Exp. Date-** Dec. 2011 **M.R.P.-** Rs. 24.00 (Inclusive of all taxes) **Mfd. By:** YAVI PHARMA KANPUR ROAD, LUCKNOW UP- 226001

2. Lemon Syrup BP

It is an extemporaneous preparation. Lemon Syrup BP has a weight per ml of about 1.33 g and the content of citric acid monohydrate, $(C_6H_8O_7.H_2O)$ is 2.2-2.6% w/v.

Composition	Method of preparation
Lemon spirit- 5 ml Citric acid monohydrate-25 g Invert syrup-100 ml Syrup q.s.-1000 ml	Dissolve the citric acid monohydrate in some amount of the syrup then add the invert syrup and the lemon spirit gradually. Add sufficient quantity of syrup to produce the final volume to 1000 ml and mix.

Label

LEMON SYRUP BP (50 ml)		
Composition: Each 50 ml contains, Lemon spirit- 0.25 ml Citric acid monohydrate- 1.25 g Invert syrup- 5 ml Syrup q.s.- 50 ml **Dose :** 15 ml **Storage:** Store in airtight, light-resistant container in cool place.	**LEMSYR** (Syrup) (Used as a source of vitamin C) **PROTECT FROM SUN LIGHT AND HEAT** **SHAKE WELL BEFORE USE**	**Mfg. Lic. No.-** 5G/2010 **Batch No.-** JK 0102 **Mfg. Date-** Mar. 2011 **Exp. Date-** Feb. 2012 **M.R.P.-** Rs. 24.00 (Inclusive of all taxes) **Mfd. By:** YAVI PHARMA KANPUR ROAD, LUCKNOW UP- 226001

3. Black Currant Syrup BP

The content of ascorbic acid, ($C_6H_8O_6$) is not less than 0.055% w/w and weight per ml is 1.27 to 1.30 g. Black Currant Syrup BP contains about 7.5 mg of ascorbic acid per 10 ml. The requirement for content of ascorbic acid does not apply when Black Currant Syrup BP is used as a flavoring agent for pharmaceutical purposes.

Composition	Method of Preparation
Sucrose- 700 g Clarified juice of Black Currant or Concentrated Black Currant juice- 560 ml Benzoic acid- q.s. Permitted food grade colors- q.s.	Dissolve 700 g of sucrose either in 560 ml of clarified juice, previously diluted with water to a weight per ml of 1.045 g, or in 560 ml of a solution of the same weight per ml prepared from the concentrated juice of commerce and water, and adding to this solution sufficient benzoic acid to give a final concentration of not more than 800 ppm, or sufficient sodium metabisulphite or other suitable sulphite to give a final concentration of not more than 350 ppm of sulphur dioxide.

Label

<table>
<tr><td colspan="3" style="text-align:center;">BLACK CURRANT SYRUP BP
(50 ml)</td></tr>
<tr>
<td>Composition:

Each 50 ml contains,

Lemon spirit- 0.25 ml

Citric acid monohydrate- 1.25 g

Invert syrup- 5 ml

Syrup q.s.- 50 ml

Dose : 15 ml

Storage: Store in well-filled, light-resistant container in cool place.</td>
<td style="text-align:center;">YAVISYR

(Syrup)

(Used as flavouring and sweetening agent)

PROTECT FROM SUN LIGHT AND HEAT

SHAKE WELL BEFORE USE</td>
<td>Mfg. Lic. No.- 2D/2010

Batch No.- SD 0230

Mfg. Date- Apr. 2011

Exp. Date- Mar. 2012

M.R.P.- Rs. 22.00

(Inclusive of all taxes)

Mfd. By: YAVI PHARMA

KANPUR ROAD, LUCKNOW

UP- 226001</td>
</tr>
</table>

4. Tolu Balsam Syrup USP

Tolu Balsam is oleo-resin which is obtained from *Myroxylon balsamam* (Family-Leguminosae). It contains 25-50% of free or combined acids, expressed as cinnamic acid ($C_9H_8O_2$).

Composition	Method of Preparation
Tolu balsam tincture- 50 ml Magnesium carbonate- 10 g Sucrose- 820 g Purified water q.s.- 1000 ml	(A) Add the tincture all at once to the magnesium carbonate and 60 g of sucrose in a mortar and mix. Gradually add 430 ml of purified water with trituration and filter. Dissolve the remainder of the sucrose in the clear filtrate with gentle heating. Strain the syrup while warm and add sufficient purified water through the strainer to make the product 1000 ml and mix. (B) Put 760 g of sucrose in a suitable percolator. The neck of which is nearly filled with loosely packed cotton, moistened after packing with a few drops of water. Pour the filtrate on the sucrose and regulate the outflow to a steady drip of percolate. When all of the liquid has run through, return the portions of the percolate, if any, to dissolve all the sucrose. Then pass enough purified water through the cotton to make the product 1000 ml and mix.

Label

TOLU BALSAM SYRUP USP (50 ml)		
Composition: Each 50 ml contains, Tolu balsam tincture- 2.5 ml Sucrose- 41 g Purified water q.s.- 50 ml **Storage-** Store in tight containers at controlled room temperature.	**TOLBAL-SYR** (Syrup) (Used as expectorant) **PROTECT FROM SUN LIGHT AND HEAT** **SHAKE WELL BEFORE USE**	**Mfg. Lic. No.-** 3J/2010 **Batch No.-** CD 0254 **Mfg. Date-** May 2011 **Exp. Date-** Apr. 2011 **M.R.P.-** Rs. 30.00 (Inclusive of all taxes) **Mfd. By:** YAVI PHARMA KANPUR ROAD, LUCKNOW UP- 226001

5. Salbutamol Sulphate Syrup IP

Salbutamol Sulphate Syrup IP contains Salbutamol Sulphate equivalent to not less than 90% and not more than 110% of the stated amount of salbutamol ($C_{13}H_{21}NO_3$). The usual strength is equivalent of 2 mg of salbutamol in 5 ml (1 mg of salbutamol sulphate is approximately equivalent to 830 mg of salbutamol). It has pH between 3.4 and 4.5. The label of Salbutamol Sulphate Syrup IP should state the strength in terms of the equivalent amount of salbutamol in a suitable dose-volume.

Composition	Method of Preparation
Salbutamol sulphate- 0.04 g Flavoured syrup base q.s.- 100 ml	Weigh the required quantity of salbutamol sulphate, dissolve in flavored syrup base and make up the volume upto 100 ml.

Label

SALBUTAMOL SULPHATE SYRUP IP (50 ml)		
Composition: Each 50 ml contains, Salbutamol sulphate- 0.02 g Flavoured syrup base q.s.- 50 ml **Dose:** 5 to 10 ml **Storage:** Store in tightly-closed, light-resistant container in a cool place.	**SALBU-SYR** (Syrup) (Used as antiasthmatic and bronchodilator) **PROTECT FROM SUN** **LIGHT AND HEAT** **SHAKE WELL BEFORE USE**	**Mfg. Lic. No.-** 6G/2010 **Batch No.-** HN 0134 **Mfg. Date-** June 2011 **Exp. Date-** May 2012 **M.R.P.-** Rs. 25.00 (Inclusive of all taxes) **Mfd. By:** YAVI PHARMA KANPUR ROAD, LUCKNOW UP- 226001

6. Ferrous Sulphate Syrup USP

Ferrous Sulphate Syrup USP contains not less than 3.75 g and not more than 4.25 g of ferrous sulphate ($FeSO_4.7H_2O$), equivalent to not less than 0.75 g and not more than 0.85 g of elemental iron in each 100 ml of syrup. The label of this syrup should state the syrup in terms of the ferrous sulphate ($FeSO_4.7H_2O$), and in terms of the content of elemental iron.

Composition	Method of Preparation
Ferrous sulphate- 40 g Citric acid (Hydrous) 2.1 g Peppermint spirit- 2 ml Sucrose- 825 g Purified water q.s. 1000 ml	Dissolve the required quantity of ferrous sulphate, citric acid (hydrous), peppermint spirit and sucrose (200 g) in 450 ml of purified water and filter the solution until clear. Dissolve the remainder of the sucrose (625 g) in the clear filtrate and add purified water sufficient to make 1000 ml. Mix and filter, if necessary through a pledget of cotton.

Label

FERROUS SULPHATE SYRUP USP **(50 ml)**		
Composition: Each 50 ml contains, Ferrous sulphate- 2 g Citric acid (Hydrous) 0.1 g Peppermint spirit- 0.1 ml Sucrose- 41.25 g Purified water q.s.- 50 ml **Storage:** Store in tight container in cool place.	**FERRSUL-SYR** (Syrup) (Used as a source of iron) **PROTECT FROM SUN** **LIGHT AND HEAT** **SHAKE WELL BEFORE USE**	**Mfg. Lic. No.-** 2L/2010 **Batch No.-** MN 0322 **Mfg. Date-** Jan. 2011 **Exp. Date-** Dec. 2011 **M.R.P.-** Rs. 34.00 (Inclusive of all taxes) **Mfd. By:** YAVI PHARMA KANPUR ROAD, LUCKNOW UP- 226001

Marketed preparations

Active Ingredient(s)	Marketed Preparation (Manufacturer)
Ibuprofen	**FEBRILIX** (ABBOTT)
Ibuprofen and Paracetamol	**MAGADOL** (ALEMBIC)
Paracetamol	**37-C** (AGRON REMEDIES), **ANMOL** (NAC INTERNATIONAL), **CROCIN** (GLAXO-SMITHKLINE), **DISPAR** (REKVINA), **FEBREX** (INDOCO), **LEXIMOL** (LEXICON BIOTECH), **METACIN** (THEMIS PHARMA), **PARACIN** (STADMED), **PARA-HL** (H.L.HEALTH CARE), **PARATOP** (HEALER'S LAB), **ULTRAGIN** (WYETH), **THERMOL** (BAL PHARMA), **PYRIGESIC** (EAST INDIA)

Table Contd...

Active Ingredient(s)	Marketed Preparation (Manufacturer)
Carbamazepine	**TEGRITAL** (NOVARTIS)
Nimesulide	**AGRANIM** (AGRAWAL PHARMA), **NEMTAB** (HEALER'S LAB), **NIMELID** (COSMAS PHARMA), **NIMUTAL** (COSTAL HEALTHCARE), **NIPIN** (LACQURE H.CARE)
Isoniazid and Vit. B_6	**SIOZIDE** (ALBERT DAVID)
Ampicillin and Cloxacillin	**BILACTAM** (CFL), **DUOCLOX** (FDC), **ELCLOX** (ELDER)
Amoxycillin	**AD-MOX** (BIO-SWISS PHARMA), **AMOXIL** (GERMAN REMEDIES), **AMOXIVAN** (KHANDELWAL), **ARISTROMOX** (ARISTRO), **DYNAMOX** (MICRO LAB), **LINMOX** (AJANTA PHARMA)
Cefixime	**AB-CEF** (BESTOCHEM), **ALTIDOR** (VSAAR PHARMA), **AMOXIM** (AMOR PHARMA), **BACIFER** (SYMBIOSIS L.SCIENCES), **CEFINOVA** (INNOVA)
Chloramphenicol	**ENTEROMYCETIN** (DEYS), **PARAXIN** (NICHOLAS)
Azithromycin	**AZIFECT** (EFFECT BIOTECH), **AZIFIX** (SERVE H.CARE), **AZIFORCE** (BIOWIN CHEMICALS), **AZILA** (ALPHA LAB), **AZITHRAL** (ALEMBIC)
Chloroquine	**APAQUINE** (AGRAWAL PHARMA), **ARQUIN** (AGRON), **LAQUIN** (STADMED), **LARIAGO** (IPCA), **PARAQUIN DS** (SHREYA), **QUINOWIN** (TAURUS LAB), **QUINROSS** (MERIND), **REOCHIN** (BAYER)
Ribavirin	**RIBAVIN** (LUPIN), **VIRAZIDE** (LUPIN)
Lamivudine	**LAMIVIR** (CIPLA)
Albendazole	**ABWORM** (ATHENS LABS), **AH-1** (OBSURGE BIOTECH), **ALBANZ** (NATURE ANDTIME), **ALBENDA** (ALPHA LAB), **ALBOM** (OM BIOTECH), **ALBOND** (HIMSAGAR LABS), **NOWORM** (ALKEM)
Diethyl carbamazine	**BANOCIDE** (GLAXO-SMITHKLINE), **HETRAZAN** (WYETH)
Domperidone	**DOMCOLIC** (ZYDUS CADILA), **DOMKAIR** (PDC H.CARE), **MOTINORM** (MEDLEY)
Promethazine	**ALLERZINE** (OYSTER LABS)
Promethazine and Paracetamol	**BIODOL-P** (ULTRAMARK H. CARE), **NIMKAIR-F** (PDC H. CARE), **PARAMAX-P** (BESTOCHEM), **PROSIP** (HELAX H. CARE), **PROSYM-P** (SYMBIOSIS LAB), **WELCOF-P** (COSMAS), **ZYMOL** (ARMOUR)

Table *Contd...*

Active Ingredient(s)	Marketed Preparation (Manufacturer)
Phenobarbitone	**BARBINOL** (HUMAN ANTIBIOTIC PHARMA), **EPIREST** (UNICURE INDIA), **GARDENAL** (NICHOLAS)
Sodium valproate	**ENCORATE** (SUN PHARMA), **VALPROL** (INTAS)
Piracetam	**ANTAM** (ANANT PHARMA), **ARKACETAM** (RKG PHARMA), **BRENTOR** (CONCORD), **CETAM** (TAURUS LAB), **EVITAM** (SWISS BIOLABS), **NORMABRAIN** (TORRENT), **PENTOR** (JPEE DRUGS), **PIRAMENT** (INNOVA)
Mecobalamin	**MBZ** (ALCARE LAB), **COBADAY** (GENPAX), **MECOTECH** (NUTRAMAX HERBALS), **MODICOBAL PLUS** (MODI PHARMA)
Magaldrate	**ALFACID** (ALFAPHARMA), **DIGESTY** (ATHENS LABS), **PEROGEL** (JPEE DRUGS), **ROLAC** (WYETH)
Codeine	**COREX** (PFIZER), **CODOKUFF** (GERMAN REMEDIES), **CODYCIP** (UNIQUE LIFE SCIENCES)

EXERCISE - 6

Object

To prepare and submit 50 ml Simple Syrup BP.

Theory

Syrups are aqueous preparations characterized by a sweet taste and a viscous consistency. Syrups usually contain aromatic or other flavoring agents. Each dose from a multidose container is administered by means of a device suitable for measuring the prescribed volume. The device is usually a spoon or a cup for volume of 5 ml or multiples thereof. Simple Syrup BP has optical rotation +56° to +60° and weight per ml is 1.315 to 1.333 g. It is an extemporaneous preparation.

Syrup BP contains 66.7% w/w of sucrose as the solute in 33.3% w/w of water as the solvent. Simple syrups do not contain active ingredients. They are not intended to be administered as such but are used as vehicle for their flavoring and sweetening properties. Syrups should be freshly prepared unless they contain suitable antimicrobial preservatives.

Formula

Ingredients	Quantity Required
Sucrose	667 g
Preservatives	q.s.
Purified water q.s. to	1000 g

Apparatus

Glass beaker, measuring cylinder and volumetric pipette.

Procedure

Weigh the required quantity of sucrose and heat sucrose with purified water together until dissolved. Afterward shake occasionally then add sufficient boiling purified water to produce 1000 g. If necessary filter the syrup. Transfer in clean, dried amber colored glass container and close it tightly.

Category

Pharmaceutical aid.

Dose

15 to 30 ml

Therapeutic Use

Simple Syrup BP is used as sweetening agent.

Storage

Simple Syrup BP should be stored in well-closed, light resistant container in cool place. Syrup should not be exposed to undue fluctuations in temperature. It should be stored at temperatures not exceeding 30°C.

Label

The label should state (1) the date after which the syrup is not intended to be used; (2) the conditions under which the syrup should be stored. The label should also state the names and proportions of any added antimicrobial preservatives. When antimicrobial preservatives are added the suitability of the syrup as a vehicle or diluent should be confirmed before use. The pH of syrup may affect the solubility of basic or acidic materials.

The label should have the caution 'PROTECT FROM SUN LIGHT' and 'SHAKE WELL BEFORE USE' in red ink.

Caution

Fill the cool syrup in the bottle at room temperature or if hot syrup is filled in the bottle, it should be occasionally shaken until it reaches the room temperature otherwise condensate water molecule may dilute the upper layer of the syrup, which causes fermentation.

Specimen Label

The specimen label for Simple Syrup BP is given as:

<table>
<tr><td colspan="3" align="center">SIMPLE SYRUP BP
(50 ml)</td></tr>
<tr>
<td>Composition:
Each 50 ml contains,
Sucrose- 33.35 g
Purified water q.s.- 50 ml
Dose: 15 to 30 ml
Storage: Store in well-closed, light-resistant container in cool place.</td>
<td align="center">SIMSYRUP
(Syrup)
(Used as sweetening agent and vehicle)

SHAKE WELL BEFORE USE
PROTECT FROM SUN LIGHT</td>
<td>Mfg. Lic. No.- 5M/2010
Batch No.- NC 0564
Mfg. Date- Oct. 2011
Exp. Date- Sep. 2012
M.R.P.- Rs. 25.00
(Inclusive of all taxes)
Mfd. By: YAVI PHARMA
KANPUR ROAD, LUCKNOW
UP- 226001</td>
</tr>
</table>

EXERCISE - 7

Object

To prepare and submit 50 ml Simple Syrup USP/NF.

Theory

Syrup is essentially sugar dissolved in water, with or without flavors. The syrup employed as a base for medicinal purposes consists of a concentrated or saturated solution of refined sugar in distilled water. Therapeutic agents may either be directly incorporated into these systems or may be added when the syrup is being prepared. If the former method is employed, it is important to ensure that the therapeutic agent is soluble within the syrup base.

The choice of syrup vehicle must be performed with due consideration to the physicochemical properties of the therapeutic agent. For example, cherry syrup and orange syrup are acidic and therefore the solubility of acidic or some zwitterionic therapeutic agents may be lowered and may result in precipitation of the drug substance. Under these circumstances, the physical stability of the preparation will have been compromised and the shelf-life of the product will have been exceeded.

The use of acidic syrups may additionally result in reduced chemical stability for acid-labile therapeutic agents. Oral syrups should not be too acidic, to enhance palatability. Packaging may also be susceptible: undue alkalinity will attack glass container.

Formula

Ingredients	Quantity Required
Sucrose	647.4 g
Purified water q.s. to	1000 g

Or

Ingredients	Quantity Required
Sucrose	850 g
Purified water q.s. to	1000 ml

Apparatus

Glass beaker, measuring cylinder, volumetric pipette and percolator.

Procedure

Simple syrup USP/NF is prepared by percolation method. In this method, the required quantity of sucrose is measured and placed in a suitable percolator, and purified water is allowed to pass slowly through the sucrose. The neck of the percolator is packed with cotton. For complete dissolution of sucrose, the percolate is returned back to the percolator. Cotton plug and inside of the percolator should be rinsed with purified water. Final volume is adjusted by adding more purified water. The final product should be transferred in clean amber colored glass container and closed tightly.

Category

Pharmaceutical aid.

Dose

15 to 30 ml

Therapeutic Use

Simple syrups are used as vehicles. Their sweet taste causes them to be a preferred form for the administration of bitter and nauseating drugs.

Storage

Simple syrup USP/NF should be stored in well-closed, light resistant container in cool place.

Label

The label should have the direction 'SHAKE WELL BEFORE USE' and the caution 'PROTECT FROM SUN LIGHT AND HEAT' in red ink. The label should also state (1) the date after which the syrup is not intended to be used, and (2) the conditions under which the syrup should be stored.

Specimen Label

The specimen label for Simple Syrup USP/NF is given as:

<table>
<tr><td colspan="3" align="center">SIMPLE SYRUP USP/NF
(50 ml)</td></tr>
<tr>
<td>Composition:
Each 50 ml contains,
Sucrose- 32.37 g
Purified water q.s.- 50 ml
Dose- 15 to 30 ml
Storage- Store in well-closed, light-resistant container in cool place.</td>
<td align="center">SISYRUP
(Syrup)
(Used as sweetening agent and vehicle)

SHAKE WELL BEFORE USE
PROTECT FROM SUN LIGHT</td>
<td>Mfg. Lic. No.- 2D/2010
Batch No.- UK 0112
Mfg. Date- Sep. 2011
Exp. Date- Aug. 2012
M.R.P.- Rs. 27.00
(Inclusive of all taxes)
Mfd. By: YAVI PHARMA
KANPUR ROAD, LUCKNOW
UP- 226001</td>
</tr>
</table>

EXERCISE - 8

Object

To prepare and submit 50 ml Simple Syrup IP.

Theory

Syrups are highly concentrated, aqueous solutions of sucrose or a sugar substitute that traditionally contain a flavoring agent, e.g. cherry syrup, cocoa syrup, orange syrup, raspberry syrup. An unflavored syrup is available that is composed of an aqueous solution containing high percentage of sucrose.

Simple Syrup IP is a concentrated or nearly saturated solution of sucrose in purified water. It contains 66.7% w/w sucrose. At such concentration, the solubility of sucrose is slow. Therefore to increase the solubility of sucrose, the Simple Syrup IP is prepared by the application of heat.

Sucrose is partially hydrolyzed in to dextrose (glucose) and levulose (fructose). These monosaccharides are known as Invert sugars. The inversion of sucrose is confirmed by measuring its optical rotation. Syrup should be always dispensed in dry bottles because moisture present in the wet bottle may cause fermentation. Simple Syrup IP has density 1.313 at 20°C.

Formula

Ingredients	Quantity Required
Sucrose	667 g
Purified water q.s. to	1000 g

Apparatus

Glass beaker, measuring cylinder and volumetric pipette.

Procedure

Measure the required quantity of sucrose and heat sucrose with purified water together until dissolved. Afterward shake occasionally then add sufficient boiling purified water to produce 1000 g. Transfer in clean, dry, amber colored, narrow mouthed glass container and close it tightly with plastic screw cap.

Category

Pharmaceutical aid.

Dose

15 to 30 ml

Therapeutic Use

Simple Syrup IP is used as sweet vehicle in the preparations containing bitter and nauseous substances. It has high osmotic pressure, which prevents the growth of microorganisms and serves as a preservative. It can also be used as the base for various flavored and medicinal syrups. Syrups are also used in the manufacture of other preparations, such as mixtures or elixirs. Syrup and glycerol, which are used in oral emulsions as sweetening agents, will increase the viscosity of the continuous phase.

Storage

Simple Syrup IP should be stored in well-closed, light resistant container in cool place. If syrup is prepared in large quantity, then it should be always stored in loosely stoppered glass bottle because if fermentation takes place, CO_2 gas will liberate, which increase the pressure inside the bottle and may lead to bursting of the bottle.

Label

The label should have the direction 'SHAKE WELL BEFORE USE' and 'PROTECT FROM SUN LIGHT AND HEAT' printed in red ink.

Caution

The use of heat facilitates rapid solution of sugar but excessive heating leads to the inversion of sucrose and hydrolyzed into monosaccharide dextrose and fructose. The colorless syrup darkens due to the effect of heat on the levulose portion of invert sugar.

The cool syrup should be filled in the bottle at room temperature or if hot syrup is filled in the bottle it should be occasionally shaked until it reaches to the room temperature otherwise condensate water molecule may dilute the upper layer of the syrup which causes fermentation.

Specimen Label

The specimen label for Simple Syrup IP is given as:

<table>
<tr><td colspan="3" align="center">SIMPLE SYRUP IP
(50 ml)</td></tr>
<tr>
<td>Composition:
Each 50 ml contains,
Sucrose- 33.35 g
Purified water q.s.- 50 ml
Dose: 15 to 30 ml
Storage: Store in well-closed, light-resistant container in cool place.</td>
<td align="center">SIMPSYRUP
(Syrup)
(Used as sweetening agent, preservative and vehicle)

SHAKE WELL BEFORE USE PROTECT FROM SUN LIGHT</td>
<td>Mfg. Lic. No.- 2K/2010
Batch No.- DC 0241
Mfg. Date- Nov. 2011
Exp. Date- Oct. 2012
M.R.P.- Rs. 25.00
(Inclusive of all taxes)
Mfd. By: YAVI PHARMA
KANPUR ROAD, LUCKNOW
UP- 226001</td>
</tr>
</table>

CHAPTER 4

ELIXIRS

Elixirs became popular in mid-nineteenth century. The word is derived apparently from the Arabic *al-iksir*, which is an Arabic form of the Greek, *xirion*. Originally the term meant "dry powder." Elixir Rubrum, one of the most renowned alchemical compounds, could supposedly turn mercury to gold or prolong life. The European elixirs were generally bitter. One of the first American elixirs was Cordial Elixir of Quinine (ca. 1838), made by John T. Heinitsh.

Elixirs are aromatic, sweetened hydroalcoholic solutions containing medicinal substances. They are liquids having an aromatic odor and a pleasant taste in order to mask an unpleasant taste of medicament and can be taken orally to cure one's ills. The color of elixirs varies according to the nature of the ingredients; some are artificially colored. When used as a pharmaceutical preparation, it contains an active ingredient (such as morphine) which is dissolved in a solution of ethyl alcohol (usually 40-60%).

Elixirs can be categorized into two classes- Non-medicated and Medicated elixirs. **Nonmedicated elixirs** are used as vehicles like Aromatic Elixir USP while **medicated elixirs** are used for the therapeutic effect of the medicament which they contain like Phenobarbital Elixir BP, Piperazine Citrate Elixir BP, Chlorpheniramine Maleate Elixir USP.

Elixirs are usually less sweet and less viscous than syrups and may contain less or no sucrose. Since elixirs contain a lower proportion of sugar, they are consequently less effective than syrups in masking the taste of drugs. In contrast to aqueous syrups, elixirs are better able to maintain both water soluble and alcohol-soluble components in solution due to their hydroalcoholic properties. These stable characteristics often make elixirs preferable to syrups.

All elixirs contain flavoring and coloring agents to enhance their palatability and appearance. Elixirs containing over 10-12% alcohol are usually self-preserving and do not require the addition of antimicrobial agents for preservation. Alcohol precipitates tragacanth, acacia, agar and inorganic salts from aqueous solutions; therefore such substances should either be absent from the aqueous phase or present in such low concentrations so as not to promote precipitation on standing. Examples of some commonly used elixirs include Dexamethasone Elixir USP, Pentobarbital Elixir USP, Diphenhydramine HCl Elixir and Digoxin Elixir.

Elixir is strictly a solution of a potent or nauseous drug. If the active agent is sensitive to moisture, it may be formulated as a flavored powder or granulation and then simply dissolved in water immediately prior to administration.

Components of Elixir

The typical components of an elixir are as follow:

(a) Purified Water

(b) Alcohol

The concentration of alcohol required in the elixir is unique to each formulation and is sufficient to ensure that all of the other components within the formulation remain in solution. The concentration of alcohol varies depending on the formulation. Generally the concentration of alcohol is greater than 10% v/v; however, in some preparations, the concentration of alcohol may be greater than 40% v/v. The presence of alcohol in elixirs provides following advantages,

(i)   Alcohol enhances the solubility of a drug,

(ii) It prevents the growth of microorganisms, and

(iii) If the quantity of alcohol is more than 20% in the preparation then there is no need of extra preservatives.

(c) Polyol Co-solvents

Polyol co-solvents, e.g. propylene glycol, glycerol, may be employed in pharmaceutical elixirs to enhance the solubility of the therapeutic agent and associated excipients. The inclusion of these ingredients enables the concentration of alcohol to be reduced.

As before, the concentration of co-solvents employed is dependent on the concentration of alcohol present, the type of co-solvent used and the solubility of the other ingredients in the alcohol/co-solvent blend.

(d) Sweetening Agents

The concentration of sucrose in elixirs is less than that in syrups and accordingly elixirs require the addition of sweetening agents. The types of sweetening agents used are similar to those used in syrups, namely syrup, sorbitol solution and artificial sweeteners such as saccharin sodium.

We must remember that the high concentration of alcohol prohibits the incorporation of high concentrations of sucrose due to the limited solubility of this sweetening agent in the elixir vehicle. This problem can be easily solved by saccharin sodium, a sweetening agent which is used in small quantities and which exhibits the required solubility profile in the elixir, is employed.

(e) Flavors and Colors

All pharmaceutical elixirs contain flavors and colors to increase the palatability and enhance the aesthetic qualities of the formulation. The presence of alcohol in the formulation allows the pharmaceutical scientist to use flavors and colors that may perhaps exhibit inappropriate solubility in aqueous solution. The selected color should optimally match the chosen flavor.

(f) Preservatives

Due to the antimicrobial properties of this co-solvent, preservatives are not required in pharmaceutical elixirs that contain greater than about 12% v/v alcohol.

(g) Viscosity Modifiers

The addition of viscosity-enhancing agents, e.g. hydrophilic polymers, may be required to optimize the rheological properties of elixirs.

Some elixirs are also available in granules or powder forms because certain active ingredients are unstable in solution form e.g. phenoxy methyl penicillin. These types of elixirs are prepared by adding measured quantity of water and shaken up until a solution is complete. These elixirs should be used within one week after their reconstitution and stored in well closed container in cool place.

Methods of Preparation

Simple solution is the general process employed in preparing elixirs. Many are prepared, however, by adding the medicinal substances directly to aromatic elixir, which is an elixir-base. While elixirs are very simple to mix, it should be noted that most elixirs are very difficult to filter, and since most elixirs require filtration, filtration by suction is the recommended method.

The simple method of preparation of elixir comprises the dissolution of ingredients with agitation or admixture of two or more liquid components in a suitable solvent. Usually alcohol soluble substances are dissolved in alcohol and aqueous soluble in water separately. The aqueous solution is then added to the alcoholic solution with constant stirring and the volume made up with solvent specified in the formulation. At this time the formulation may not be clear due to the separation of some of the flavoring agents. In such a condition elixir is allowed to stand for some time to ensure the saturation of the hydroalcoholic solvent and allowing the oil globules to coalesce. Talc or some other absorbents can be used to absorb the excess of the oil and assist in their removal from solution. Filtration gives a clear product.

For example, USP/NF method of preparation of Simple Elixir includes Compound Spirit of Orange (12 ml), syrup (375 ml), precipitated calcium phosphate (15 g), deodorized alcohol, and distilled water in a sufficient quantity to make 1000 ml. To the Compound Spirit of Orange enough deodorized alcohol is added to make 250 ml. To this solution add the syrup in several portions, agitating after each addition, and afterwards add, in the same manner (375 ml) of distilled water. Mix the precipitated calcium phosphate intimately with the liquid, and then filter through a wetted filter, returning the first portions of the filtrate until a transparent liquid is obtained. Lastly, wash the filter with a mixture of deodorized alcohol and distilled water (1:3 volume), until the product measures 1000 ml.

General Steps Involved in Preparation of Elixirs

1. Elixirs are prepared by simple solution method by dissolving the alcohol soluble substances in alcohol and water soluble substances in water.
2. Add aqueous solution to the alcoholic solution with continuous stirring to avoid the formation of precipitate.
3. When two solutions are completely mixed make up the final volume with vehicle. If final mixture obtained is not clear, then allow the preparation to stand for few hours for complete saturation of hydroalcoholic vehicle and to permit the oil globules of volatile oil to coalesce.
4. To remove undissolved oil, purified talc (3-5%) is added to the preparation as a filter aid, which adsorbs excessive amount of oil and removes them from the preparation after final filtration. The filter paper should be wetted with the hydroalcoholic solution of the same alcoholic strength.
5. The collection flask should be either completely dried or rinsed with same hydroalcoholic vehicle that is used for the preparation for the elixirs.

Therapeutic Uses

Non medicated elixirs are generally employed as flavoring agents while medicated elixirs are used for the therapeutic effect of the drug which they contain. For example, Chloral hydrate Elixir (200 mg/5 ml) is used for pre-operative sedation. Aromatic Elixir USP is a carminative but generally employed as a flavoring agent.

Promethazine hydrochloride Elixir (5 mg/5 ml) is a sedative antihistamine. It is used as premedication prior to surgery. It is also used as antiemetic in nausea, vomiting, labyrinthine disorders and in motion sickness.

Chlorphenamine maleate Elixir (2 mg/5 ml) is a sedative antihistamine and is used in symptomatic relief of allergy, allergic rhinitis (hay fever), conjunctivitis, urticaria, insect stings and pruritus of allergic origin. It is used as adjunct in the emergency treatment of anaphylactic shock and severe angioedema.

Phenobarbital Elixir (15 mg/5 ml) is used in generalized tonic-clonic seizures, febrile convulsions and status epilepticus.

Piperazine citrate Elixir IP expels the round worms and thread worms from the intestine so this elixir is used as anthelmintic.

Paracetamol Paediatric Elixir IP is used as analgesic and antipyretic for children. Paediatric Chloral Hydrate Elixir BP is most widely used as sedative for inducing sleep in children. Terpine Hydrate Elixir IP is used as expectorant.

Dose

The recommended dose of most of the elixirs is 5 to 10 ml. The dosage is usually taken using a 5 ml medicine spoon, although smaller volumes can be given using a volumetric dropper.

Storage Conditions

Since elixirs contain alcohol and some volatile oils, which may deteriorate in presence of air and light, therefore elixirs should be stored in tightly closed, light resistant containers and in a cool place.

Specific Labeling Requirement

Due to the presence of alcohol and other volatile constituents and to avoid their degradation from sun light, the label of elixirs should have the caution 'PROTECT FROM SUN LIGHT'.

Contraindications

Elixirs have high content of ethyl alcohol so elixirs should not be given to the paediatric patients and to those adults who want to avoid alcohol. Medicated elixirs like Promethazine Hydrochloride Elixir are contraindicated for child under 1 year, in impaired consciousness due to cerebral depressants or of other origin and in porphyria. Chlorphenamine Maleate Elixir is contraindicated in prostatic enlargement, urinary retention, ileus or pyloric stenosis, glaucoma and for child under 1 year.

Examples of Some Elixirs

1. Phenobarbital Elixir BP

Phenobarbital Elixir BP is an oral solution containing 0.3% w/v of phenobarbital in a suitable flavored vehicle containing a sufficient volume of ethanol (96%) or of an appropriate dilute ethanol to give a final concentration of 38% v/v of ethanol. The content of Phenobarbital varies from 0.27 to 0.33% w/v. Phenobarbital Elixir BP has ethanol content of 36 to 40% v/v.

Glycerin is often added to enhance the solubility of phenobarbital. The elixir is commonly sweetened with syrup, flavored with orange oil and colored red with an approved colorant.

Composition	Method of Preparation	Caution
Phenobarbital- 0.4 g Orange oil- 0.025 ml Propylene glycol- 10 ml Alcohol- 20 ml Sorbitol solution- 60 ml Color- q.s. Purified water q.s. to- 100 ml	Dissolved the ingredients in their respective solvents e.g. alcohol soluble ingredients in alcohol and water soluble ingredients in purified water. Then mixed the solutions. Talc was added to absorb excess oil and filtered it.	To avoid the precipitation of alcohol soluble ingredients, the aqueous solution is always added to alcoholic solution.

Label

PHENOBARBITAL ELIXIR BP (50 ml)		
Composition: Each 50 ml contains, Phenobarbital- 0.2 g Propylene glycol- 5 ml Alcohol- 10 ml Sorbitol solution- 30 ml Color- q.s. Purified water q.s. to- 50 ml **Dose:** 7 to 30 ml/day	**PHENOLIXIR** (Elixir) (Used as a sedative and hypnotic) **PROTECT FROM SUN LIGHT** Store in a well-closed container and protected from light.	**Mfg. Lic. No.-** 9E/2010 **Batch No.-** KK 0620 **Mfg. Date-** May, 2011 **Exp. Date-** Apr. 2012 **M.R.P.-** Rs. 30.00 (Inclusive of all taxes) **Mfd. By:** YAVI PHARMA KANPUR ROAD, LUCKNOW UP- 226001

2. Piperazine Citrate Elixir BP

Piperazine Citrate Elixir BP is an oral solution containing 18.75% w/v of Piperazine Citrate in a suitable flavored vehicle. The content of piperazine citrate is 15.3 to 17.7% w/v and it has weight per ml 1.20 to 1.30 g. Piperazine Citrate Elixir BP contains the equivalent of about 750 mg of piperazine hydrate in 5 ml. Piperazine Citrate Elixir BP should be protected from light.

Composition	Method of Preparation
Piperazine Citrate- 18.75 g Syrup- q.s. Ethyl alcohol- q.s. Purified water q.s.-100 ml	Dissolve piperazine citrate in purified water, other additives are added in required quantity, and finally purified water is added in sufficient quantity to produce 100 ml and mixed. On addition of purified water, the alcohol soluble but water insoluble constituents may precipitate so, if necessary, the elixir should be filtered.

Label

Composition:	PIPERALIXIR	Mfg. Lic. No.- 4H/2010
PIPERAZINE CITRATE ELIXIR BP **(50 ml)**		
Each 50 ml contains,	**PIPERALIXIR**	**Batch No.-** WS 189
Piperazine citrate- 2.5 g	(Elixir)	**Mfg. Date-** Mar, 2011
Syrup- q.s.	(Used as antihelminthic)	**Exp. Date-** Feb. 2012
Ethyl alcohol- q.s.		**M.R.P.-** Rs. 28.00
Purified water q.s.-50 ml	**PROTECT FROM SUN**	(Inclusive of all taxes)
Dose: As prescribed by physician	**LIGHT**	**Mfd. By:** YAVI PHARMA
Storage: Store in a tightly closed container.		KANPUR ROAD, LUCKNOW UP- 226001

3. Terpin Hydrate Elixir

Terpin hydrate is slightly soluble in water but soluble in alcohol. The alcohol content of the elixir is about 39 to 44% v/v.

Composition	Method of Preparation
Terpin hydrate- 5 g Orange oil- 0.2 ml Glycerin- 40 ml Syrup- 10 ml Ethyl alcohol- 42.5 ml Purified water q.s.-100 ml	Dissolve Terpin hydrate in alcohol, other additives are added in required quantity, and finally purified water is added in sufficient quantity to produce 100 ml and mixed. On addition of purified water, the alcohol soluble but water insoluble constituents may precipitate so, if necessary, the elixir should be filtered.

Label

<table>
<tr><td colspan="3" align="center">TERPIN HYDRATE ELIXIR BP
(50 ml)</td></tr>
<tr>
<td>Composition:
Each 50 ml contains,
Terpin hydrate- 2.5 g
Orange oil- 0.1 ml
Glycerin- 20 ml
Syrup- 5 ml
Ethyl alcohol- 21.25 ml
Purified water q.s.-50 ml
Dose: As directed by physician
Storage: Store in a tightly closed container.</td>
<td align="center">TERPINLIXIR
(Elixir)
(Used as an expectorant)

PROTECT FROM SUN LIGHT</td>
<td>Mfg. Lic. No.- 2C/2010
Batch No.- MH 267
Mfg. Date- Mar, 2011
Exp. Date- Feb. 2012
M.R.P.- Rs. 28.00
(Inclusive of all taxes)
Mfd. By: YAVI PHARMA KANPUR ROAD, LUCKNOW UP- 226001</td>
</tr>
</table>

4. Theophylline Elixir USP

Theophylline Elixir is a fruit-flavored reddish-orange liquid intended for oral administration, containing 80 mg of anhydrous theophylline and 20% alcohol per 15 ml. Theophylline is indicated for the treatment of the symptoms and reversible airflow obstruction associated with chronic asthma and other chronic lung diseases, e.g., emphysema and chronic bronchitis. Theophylline Elixir is contraindicated in patients with a history of hypersensitivity to theophylline or other components in the product.

Composition	Method of Preparation
Theophylline (anhydrous)- 0.53 g Syrup- 13.2 ml Sorbitol solution- 32.4 ml Alcohol- 20 ml Purified water q.s.- 100 ml	Dissolve theophylline (anhydrous) in purified water, other additives are added in required quantity, and finally purified water is added in sufficient quantity to produce 100 ml and mixed.

Label

<table>
<tr><td colspan="3" align="center">THEOPHYLLINE ELIXIR BP
(50 ml)</td></tr>
<tr>
<td>Composition:
Each 50 ml contains,
Theophylline (anhydrous) - 0.265 g
Syrup- 6.6 ml
Sorbitol solution- 16.2 ml
Alcohol- 10 ml
Purified water q.s.- 50 ml
Dose: 5 ml, 3-4 times daily
Storage: Store in a tight, light-resistant container at controlled room temperature 15°C-30°C</td>
<td align="center">THEOPHYLIXIR
(Elixir)
(Used in chronic asthma and bronchitis)

PROTECT FROM SUN LIGHT</td>
<td>Mfg. Lic. No.- 3K/2010
Batch No.- CH 115
Mfg. Date- May, 2011
Exp. Date- Mar. 2012
M.R.P.- Rs. 22.00
(Inclusive of all taxes)
Mfd. By: YAVI PHARMA KANPUR ROAD, LUCKNOW UP- 226001</td>
</tr>
</table>

5. Ephedrine Elixir BP

The content of ephedrine hydrochloride ($C_{10}H_{15}NO.HCl$) in Ephedrine Elixir BP is 0.27 to 0.33% w/v and ethanol content is 11 to 13% v/v. It is Adrenoceptor agonist.

Composition	Method of Preparation
Ephedrine hydrochloride- 0.3 g Ethanol (96%)- 12 ml Flavored syrup- 40 ml Purified water q.s.- 100 ml	Dissolve Ephedrine hydrochloride in purified water, other additives are added in required quantity, and finally purified water is added in sufficient quantity to produce 100 ml and mixed.

Label

<table>
<tr><td colspan="3" align="center">EPHEDRINE ELIXIR BP
(50 ml)</td></tr>
<tr>
<td>Composition:
Each 50 ml contains,
Ephedrine hydrochloride- 0.15 g
Ethanol (96%)- 6 ml
Flavored syrup- 20 ml
Purified water q.s.- 50 ml
Dose: 5-10 ml
Storage: Store in a tightly closed container.</td>
<td align="center">EPHELIXIR
(Elixir)
(Used as Bronchodilator)

PROTECT FROM SUN LIGHT</td>
<td>Mfg. Lic. No.- 2C/2010
Batch No.- MH 267
Mfg. Date- Mar, 2011
Exp. Date- Feb. 2012
M.R.P.- Rs. 28.00
(Inclusive of all taxes)
Mfd. By: YAVI PHARMA KANPUR ROAD, LUCKNOW UP- 226001</td>
</tr>
</table>

Marketed preparations

Active Ingredient(s)	Marketed Preparation (Manufacturer)
Bromhexine	**BROMHEXINE** (IPCA)
Theophylline	**CADIPHYLATE** (CADILA HEALTH CARE)
Ferruous sulphate	**FESOVIT ELIXIR** (GLAXO-SMITHKLINE)
Promethazine	**PHENERGAN** (NICHOLAS)
Vit B_1, B_2, B_6	**BETONIN** (ABBOTT), **BG PROT** (MERIND), **BEPLEX** (ANGLO FRENCH DRUGS)

EXERCISE - 9

Object

To prepare and submit 50 ml Aromatic Elixir USP/NF.

Theory

Elixirs are clear, flavored hydroalcoholic, sweetened liquid preparations intended for oral use. Elixirs contain one or more medicament/active ingredient, pleasant flavor, attractive color and high proportion of alcohol along with other suitable excipients including antimicrobial agents. Elixirs are more stable than mixtures due to the presence of high content of alcohol, which maintains the drug in solution.

Elixirs are less sweet and less viscous than syrups. Glycerins and syrup are used in elixirs either for increasing the solubility of medicaments or for sweetening purposes. The bitter and nauseous taste of drugs is masked up to certain limit. Due to the presence of flavoring and sweetening agents in hydroalcoholic medium, it can be easily taken by children.

Formula

Ingredients	Quantity Required
Suitable essential oil	15 ml
Syrup	375 ml
Talc	30 g
Ethanol (90%) and Purified water q.s. to	1000 ml

Apparatus

Glass beaker, measuring cylinder and volumetric pipette.

Procedure

Measure the required quantity of essential oil and dissolve in ethanol (90%) to make 250 ml. To this solution add syrup in small quantities with vigorous shaking after each addition. Afterward, in the same manner, add the required quantity of purified water to makeup the volume to 1000 ml. Mix the talc and set aside for some time. Then filter through a filter previously wetted with dilute alcohol, returning the filtrate until a clear elixir is obtained. Transfer it in a clean amber colored glass container, close it tightly and label properly.

Category

Pharmaceutical aid.

Dose

5 to 10 ml.

Therapeutic Use

Aromatic Elixir USP/NF is used for flavoring purposes and as flavored vehicle for the preparation of other pharmaceutical formulations.

Storage

Aromatic Elixir USP/NF should be stored in well-closed, light resistant container in cool place to prevent the volatilization of essential oil.

Label

The label should have the caution 'PROTECT FROM SUN LIGHT' in red ink due to the presence of volatile constituents in the preparation. The amount of alcohol content used should be mentioned on the label.

Caution

In order to maintain the highest possible alcoholic strength at all times and to avoid the separation of alcohol soluble ingredients, the alcoholic solution should not be added to the aqueous solution otherwise alcohol soluble substances will precipitate out and this precipitate is very difficult to make as diffusible.

Specimen Label

The specimen label for Aromatic Elixir USP/NF is given as:

<table>
<tr><td colspan="3" align="center">AROMATIC ELIXIR USP/NF

(50 ml)</td></tr>
<tr>
<td valign="top">

Composition:

Each 50 ml contains,

Essential oil - 0.75 ml

Syrup- 18.75 ml

Ethanol (90%) and Purified water q.s.- 50 ml

Dose- 5 to 10 ml

Storage- Store in airtight, light-resistant container in cool place.

</td>
<td valign="top" align="center">

AROLIXIR

(Aromatic Elixir)

(Flavoring agent and Vehicle)

**PROTECT FROM SUN LIGHT
NOT FOR INJECTION**

</td>
<td valign="top">

Mfg. Lic. No.- 2M/2010

Batch No.- CF 0212

Mfg. Date- Jun. 2011

Exp. Date- May 2012

M.R.P.- Rs. 23.00

(Inclusive of all taxes)

Mfd. By: YAVI PHARMA

KANPUR ROAD,
LUCKNOW UP- 226001

</td>
</tr>
</table>

CHAPTER 5

SPIRITS

Spirits are alcoholic or hydroalcoholic solutions of volatile substances prepared usually by simple solution or by admixture of the ingredients. Spirits generally contain a high concentration of alcohol e.g. Compound Orange Spirit USP contains 65 to 70% v/v alcohol and Camphor Spirit USP contains 80 to 87% v/v alcohol. Peppermint Spirit USP has alcohol content 79 to 85% v/v while Aromatic Ammonia Spirit BP has ethanol content 64 to 70% v/v. Due to more solubility of aromatic and volatile constituents in alcohol, spirits have greater concentration of these materials in solution form. Reduction of the high alcoholic content of spirits by admixture with aqueous preparations often causes turbidity.

Methods of Preparation

Depending upon the materials utilized, spirits can be prepared by following methods,

Simple Solution

Majority of the spirits are prepared by this method. In this method aromatic constituents/solutes are dissolved in alcohol by agitation. This method is used for the preparation of Chloroform Spirit and Spirit of Ether.

Solution with Maceration

This method consists of maceration of leaves of the drug in a suitable solvent to extract the desired constituents. Purified water can be used to extract the water soluble constituents. After expression, the moist macerated leaves are added to a prescribed quantity of ethyl alcohol. The volatile oil is added to the filtrate. Peppermint Spirit NF is prepared by this method.

Chemical Reaction

This method is based on the chemical reactions between the different ingredients of the spirit to enhance their solubility e.g. Aromatic Ammonia Spirit USP involves a chemical reaction converting the official ammonium carbonate to true ammonium carbonate to enhance its solubility. Ethyl Nitrite Spirit contains ethyl nitrite, which in turn, is obtained by the chemical reaction of sodium nitrite on a mixture of alcohol and sulphuric acid in cold.

Therapeutic Uses

Spirits may be used pharmaceutically as flavoring agents and preservative and medicinally for the therapeutic value of the aromatic constituent. For medicinal purposes, depending upon the particular preparation, spirits may be taken orally, can be applied externally or used by inhalation. Aromatic Ammonia Spirit BP is used as stimulant. Spirits may be used in the formulation of aromatic waters. Spirits are also used as carminative in flatulent colic.

Dose

Most of spirits are used as pharmaceutical aids (flavoring agents) e.g. Compound Orange Spirit USP, Peppermint Spirit USP and Lemon Spirit BP but for medicinal purposes, the recommended dose depends upon the particular preparation e.g. Aromatic Ammonia Spirit BP is taken as 1-5 ml diluted with water. The dose of Chloroform Spirit is 0.3-1 ml.

Storage Conditions

Spirits require storage in tight, light resistant containers to prevent loss by evaporation and to limit oxidative changes.

Specific Labeling Requirement

Since the spirits have volatile constituents, the label of spirits should have the caution 'PROTECT FROM LIGHT'. The label on the container of Spirit of Ether must have Caution: This preparation is inflammable. Keep away from naked flame. The label on the container of Industrial Methylated Spirit must indicate 'inflammable'.

Contraindication

Aromatic Ammonia Spirit BP, USP is alkaline in nature so it is incompatible with acids and salts of iron, calcium, barium and other metals and also with alkaloidal salts.

Examples of Some Spirits

1. Compound Orange Spirit USP; BP

Compound Orange Spirit USP	Compound Orange Spirit BP
It has, in each 100 ml, not less than 25 ml and not more than 30 ml of the mixed oils and it has alcohol content between 65 to 70%. **Composition:** Orange oil- 200 ml Lemon oil- 50 ml Coriander oil- 20 ml Anise oil- 5 ml Alcohol q.s.- 1000 ml **Method of preparation:** Mix the required quantity of all oils with sufficient alcohol and then add more alcohol to make the volume to 1000 ml. **Caution:** The orange oil and lemon oil having terebinthine odor should not be used in the preparation.	It has ethanol content of 86 to 90% v/v and weight per ml 0.828 to 0.841 g. **Composition:** Orange oil (terpeneless)- 2.5 ml Lemon oil (terpeneless)- 1.3 ml Anise oil- 4.25 ml Coriander oil- 6.25 ml Ethanol (90%) q.s- 1000 ml **Method of preparation:** It is prepared by simple mixing method.

Label

<table>
<tr><td colspan="3" align="center">COMPOUND ORANGE SPIRIT USP
(50 ml)</td></tr>
<tr>
<td>Composition:
Each 50 ml contains,
Orange oil- 10 ml
Lemon oil- 2.5 ml
Coriander oil- 1 ml
Anise oil- 0.25 ml
Alcohol q.s.- 50 ml
Dose: 0.3 to 1 ml
Storage: Store in tight container, protected from light in a cool place.</td>
<td align="center">ORA-SPIRIT
(Spirit)
(Used as a flavoring agent and preservative)

PROTECT FROM SUN LIGHT
NOT FOR INJECTION</td>
<td>Mfg. Lic. No.- 1V/2010
Batch No.- VM 0225
Mfg. Date- May, 2011
Exp. Date- Apr. 2012
M.R.P.- Rs. 25.00
(Inclusive of all taxes)
Mfd. By: YAVI PHARMA
KANPUR ROAD, LUCKNOW
UP- 226001</td>
</tr>
</table>

2. Peppermint Spirit USP; BP

Peppermint oil is obtained by steam distillation from the fresh over ground parts of the flowering plant of *Mentha piperita*. Peppermint oil is a colorless, pale yellow or pale greenish-yellow liquid with a characteristic odor and taste followed by a sensation of cold. It is miscible with alcohol, ether and with methylene chloride.

Peppermint Spirit USP	Peppermint Spirit BP
It contains, in each 100 ml, not less than 9 ml and not more than 11 ml of peppermint oil. It has alcohol content of 79 to 85% v/v. **Composition:** Peppermint oil- 100 ml Peppermint (coarse powder form)- 10 g Alcohol q.s. to- 1000 ml **Method of preparation:** Macerate the peppermint leaves, freed as much as possible from stems and in coarsely powdered form, for 1 hour in 500 ml of purified water and then strongly expressed them. Add the moist macerated leaves to 900 ml of alcohol and allow the mixture to stand for 6 hours with frequent agitation. Filter it and to the filtrate add the peppermint oil and alcohol to make the volume to 1000 ml.	It is an extemporaneous preparation and has ethanol content of 78 to 82% v/v and weight per ml is 0.830 to 0.840 g. **Composition:** Peppermint oil-100 ml Ethanol (90%) q.s. to- 1000 ml **Method of preparation:** Dissolve the peppermint oil in ethanol (90%) and then add sufficient ethanol (90%) to produce 1000 ml. If the solution is not clear, shake with previously sterilized purified talc and filter.

Label

PEPPERMINT SPIRIT BP (50 ml)		
Composition: Each 50 ml contains, Peppermint oil- 5 ml Ethanol (90%) q.s. to 50 ml **Dose-** 1 to 5 ml **Storage-** Store in a well-filled, airtight container, protected from light and heat.	**MINT-SPIRIT** (Spirit) (Used as a flavoring agent and preservative) **PROTECT FROM SUN LIGHT** **NOT FOR INJECTION**	**Mfg. Lic. No.-** 4H/2010 **Batch No.-** BN 0115 **Mfg. Date-** Feb. 2011 **Exp. Date-** Jan. 2012 **M.R.P.-** Rs. 20.00 (Inclusive of all taxes) **Mfd. By:** YAVI PHARMA KANPUR ROAD, LUCKNOW UP- 226001

3. Camphor Spirit USP

Camphor Spirit USP is an alcoholic solution containing not less than 9 g and not more than 11 g of camphor. It has ethanol content of 80 to 87% v/v. It should not be used by women who are pregnant or nursing and should never be applied externally to broken or burned skin.

Composition	Method of Preparation
Camphor- 100 g Ethanol q.s. to-1000 ml	Dissolve the required quantity of camphor in about 800 ml of ethanol and to this solution add more ethanol to make up the volume 1000 ml.

Label

<table>
<tr><td colspan="3" align="center">CAMPHOR SPIRIT USP
(50 ml)</td></tr>
<tr>
<td>Composition:
Each 50 ml contains,
Camphor- 5 g
Ethanol q.s. to 50 ml
Dose: 0.3 to 3.6 ml
Storage: Store in a tightly closed container and protected from light.</td>
<td align="center">CAMSPIRIT
(Spirit)
(Used as an expectorant and calming agent for the nervous system, particularly in cases of hysteria or excessive nervousness)

PROTECT FROM SUN LIGHT</td>
<td>Mfg. Lic. No.- 2C/2010
Batch No.- MH 267
Mfg. Date- Mar, 2011
Exp. Date- Feb. 2012
M.R.P.- Rs. 28.00
(Inclusive of all taxes)
Mfd. By: YAVI PHARMA KANPUR ROAD, LUCKNOW UP- 226001</td>
</tr>
</table>

4. Aromatic Ammonia Spirit USP

Aromatic Ammonia Spirit USP is a hydroalcoholic solution. It has alcohol content 62 to 68% v/v.

Composition	Method of Preparation
Ammonia- 2 g Ammonium carbonate- 4 g Alcohol- 65 ml Aromatic oils- q.s. Purified water q.s.- 100 ml	Dissolve the required quantity of ammonium carbonate in purified water, other additives are added in required quantity, and finally purified water is added in sufficient quantity to produce 100 ml and mixed.

Label

<table>
<tr><td colspan="3" align="center">**AROMATIC AMMONIA SPIRIT USP**
(50 ml)</td></tr>
<tr>
<td>**Composition:**

Each 50 ml contains,

Ammonia- 1 g

Ammonium carbonate- 2 g

Alcohol- 30.25 ml

Aromatic oils- q.s.

Purified water q.s.- 50 ml

Storage: Store in tight, light-resistant container at a temperature not exceeding 30°C.</td>
<td align="center">**AROMSPIRIT**

(Spirit)

(Used as stimulant, diuretic and diaphoretic)

PROTECT FROM SUN LIGHT</td>
<td>**Mfg. Lic. No.-** 2L/2010

Batch No.- CV 0163

Mfg. Date- May, 2011

Exp. Date- Apr. 2012

M.R.P.- Rs. 22.00
(Inclusive of all taxes)

Mfd. By: YAVI PHARMA KANPUR ROAD, LUCKNOW UP- 226001</td>
</tr>
</table>

5. Lemon Spirit BP

It has aldehydes content 3.45 to 4.6% w/v, calculated as citral and ethanol content 84 to 88% v/v and weight per ml 0.814 to 0.823 g.

Composition	Method of Preparation
Lemon oil (Terpeneless)- 100 ml Ethanol (96%) q.s. to- 1000 ml	Dissolve the required quantity of camphor in about 800 ml of ethanol and to this solution add more ethanol to make up the volume 1000 ml.

Label

<table>
<tr><td colspan="3" align="center">**LEMON SPIRIT BP**
(50 ml)</td></tr>
<tr>
<td>**Composition:**

Each 50 ml contains,
Lemon oil (Terpeneless)- 5 ml
Ethanol (96%) q.s. to- 50 ml

Storage: Store in tightly closed container and protected from light.</td>
<td align="center">**LEMSPIRIT**

(Spirit)

(Used as flavoring agent and vehicle)

PROTECT FROM SUN LIGHT</td>
<td>**Mfg. Lic. No.-** 5H/2010

Batch No.- JK 0125
Mfg. Date- Aug. 2011
Exp. Date- July 2012
M.R.P.- Rs. 22.00
(Inclusive of all taxes)

Mfd. By: YAVI PHARMA KANPUR ROAD, LUCKNOW UP- 226001</td>
</tr>
</table>

Marketed Preparations

Active Ingredient(s)	Marketed preparation (Manufacturer)
Chloroform	**CHLOROFORM SPIRIT** (K. PHARMACEUTICAL WORKS)
Aromatic Ammonia	**AMMONIA AROMATIC SPIRIT** (K. PHARMACEUTICAL WORKS)
Orange oil	**COMPOUND ORANGE SPIRIT BP** (DEOGHAR PHARMACEUTICALS)
Lemon oil	**LEMON SPIRIT BP** (DEOGHAR PHARMACEUTICALS)

EXERCISE - 10

Object

To prepare and submit 50 ml Aromatic Ammonia Spirit BP.

Theory

Spirits are alcoholic or hydroalcoholic solutions of volatile substances. Spirits are also called as essences. They generally contain higher percentage of alcohol than that in Tincture and Aromatic waters. Aromatic Ammonia Spirit BP is an extemporaneous preparation. It has the content of free ammonia 1.12 to 1.3% w/v, content of ammonium carbonate 2.76 to 3.24% w/v and ethanol content 64 to 70% v/v. Its weight per ml is 0.880 to 0.893 g.

Generally the spirits are prepared by solution method but Aromatic spirit of ammonia is prepared by distillation method because the oil of Nutmeg contains non-volatile resinous matter due to which the preparation changes to dark color on storage. In this method the distillate is collected in two portions-

First portion of distillate contains a major part of alcohol, volatile oil and small proportion of water. Second portion of distillate contains a major part of water, small proportion of alcohol and volatile oil. Second portion of distillate is heated with ammonium bicarbonate and ammonia to convert it into ammonium carbonate.

$$NH_4HCO_3 + NH_3 \longrightarrow (NH_4)_2CO_3$$

Formula

Ingredients	Quantity Required
Nutmeg oil	3 ml
Lemon oil	5 ml
Ammonium bicarbonate	25 g
Strong ammonia solution	67.5 ml
Ethanol (90%)	750 ml
Purified water q.s. to	1000 ml

Apparatus

Glass beaker, measuring cylinder, distillation flask and volumetric pipette.

Procedure

Measure the required quantity of ingredients and distil a mixture of lemon oil, nutmeg oil, ethanol (90%) and 375 ml of purified water. Reserve the first 875 ml of distillate. Distil a further 55 ml and add the ammonium bicarbonate and strong ammonia solution to the distillate. Heat on a water bath to 60°C in a sealed bottle of not less than 120 ml capacity, shaking occasionally, until solution is complete, cool, filter through absorbent cotton, mix the filtrate with the reserved distillate and add sufficient purified water to produce 1000 ml and mix. Transfer in clean amber colored glass container and close it tightly.

Caution

Lowering of the high alcoholic content of spirits by addition of aqueous preparations often causes turbidity i.e. Spirits shows incompatibility when mixed with water or with an aqueous preparation.

Specimen Label

The specimen label for Aromatic Ammonia Spirit BP is given as:

<table>
<tr><td colspan="3">AROMATIC AMMONIA SPIRIT BP
(50 ml)</td></tr>
<tr>
<td>Composition:
Each 50 ml contains,
Nutmeg oil- 0.15 ml
Lemon oil- 0.25 ml
Ammonium bicarbonate- 1.25 g
Strong ammonia solution- 3.37 ml
Ethanol (90%)- 37.5 ml
Purified water q.s.- 50 ml
Dose: 1 to 5 ml diluted with water
Storage: Store in tight, light-resistant container at a temperature not exceeding 30°C.</td>
<td>AROSPIRIT
(Spirit)
Stimulant
(Used as stimulant, diuretic and diaphoretic)

PROTECT FROM SUN LIGHT
KEEP AWAY FROM DIRECT FLAME OR FIRE</td>
<td>Mfg. Lic. No.- 5G/2010
Batch No.- KM 0502
Mfg. Date- May 2011
Exp. Date- Apr. 2012
M.R.P.- Rs. 18.00
(Inclusive of all taxes)
Mfd. By: YAVI PHARMA KANPUR ROAD, LUCKNOW UP 226001</td>
</tr>
</table>

CHAPTER 6

POWDERS

Any material ranging in particle size from 0.1 to 10000 µm may be described as powder. However, the powders used in pharmaceutical field generally have a size between 0.1 to 10 µm. The term 'powder' when in context of a dosage form describes a formulation in which a drug powder has been mixed with other powdered excipients to produce the final product. The function of the added excipients depends upon the intended use of the product. For example, coloring, flavoring and sweetening agents, may be added to powders for oral use. Thus powders are intimate mixture of dry, finely divided drug or chemicals that may be intended for internal (oral powders) or external (topical powders) use. Various physicochemical characteristics of powders are a function mainly of their size and surface area. The size of powders determines their dissolution rate, which in turn, controls the bioavailability of the drugs to the system.

Powders are one of the oldest dosage forms. They impart flexibility with regard to selection of drugs, their combination and dose; stability in case of drugs which are more stable in powdered form than in solution; rapid therapeutic effect and ease in administration to all categories of patients.

Powders show various advantages over other dosage forms. Due to greater surface area, orally administered powders of soluble medicaments have a faster dissolution rate than tablets or capsules, as these must first disintegrate before the drug dissolves. Drug absorption from such powdered preparations will therefore be faster than from the corresponding tablet or capsule, if the dissolution rate limits the rate of drug absorption. Children and those adults who experience difficulty in swallowing tablets or capsules may find powders more acceptable. Further, drugs that are too bulky to be formed into tablets or capsules of convenient size may be administered as powders. Powders are a convenient form to dispense drugs with a large dose.

Often, stability problems encountered in liquid dosage forms are avoided in powdered dosage forms. Drugs that are unstable in aqueous suspensions or solutions may be prepared in the form of powders. These are intended to be constituted by the addition of a specified quantity of water just prior to dispensing because these constituted products have limited stability; they are required to have a specified expiry date after constitution and may require storage in a refrigerator. However, the preparation of powders is time consuming and powders are not suitable dosage form for unpleasant tasting, hygroscopic and deliquescent drugs.

Oral powders are dispensed in pre-measured doses i.e. divided powders or in bulk. **Divided powders** are unit dose powders normally packed in properly folded paper and dispensed in envelopes, metal foil, or other suitable containers. However, for greater protection from the environment, the powders can be supplied by sealing individual doses in small cellophane or polyethylene envelopes i.e. small heat sealed plastic bags.

Bulk powders are the powders which are dispensed in bulk when accuracy of dosage is not critical. Bulk oral powders are limited to relatively non-potent drugs such as laxatives, antacids, dietary supplements and certain analgesics that the patient may safely measure by teaspoonful or capful. Other bulk powders include douche powders, tooth powders and dusting powders. Bulk powders are best dispensed in tight, wide-mouth glass containers for maximum protection from the atmosphere and to prevent the loss of volatile ingredients. Powders can broadly be categorized as follow:

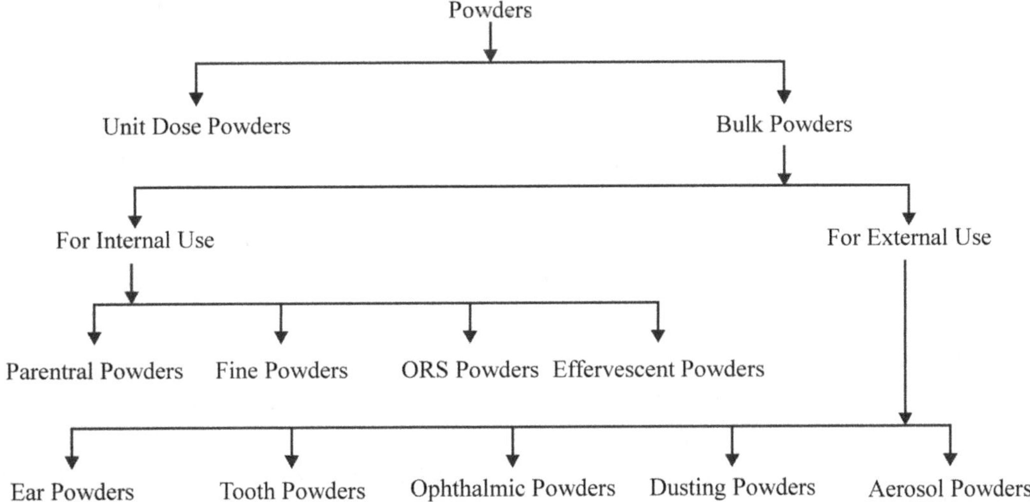

Particle Size Classification of Powders

The degree of coarseness or fineness of a powder is expressed by reference to the nominal mesh aperture size of the sieves used for measuring the size of the powders. For practical reasons, the use of sieves for measuring powder fineness for most pharmaceutical purposes is convenient but devices other than sieves must be employed for the measurement of particles less than 100 µm in nominal size. Fineness of the powder may be expressed as a % w/w passing the sieve(s) used. The following terms are used in IP-2007 for defining the particle size of powders:

1. Coarse Powder

A powder all the particles of which pass through a sieve with a nominal mesh aperture of 1,700 μm and not more than 40% by weight through a sieve with a nominal mesh aperture of 355 μm.

2. Moderately Coarse Powder

A powder all the particles of which pass through a sieve with nominal mesh aperture of 710 μm and not more than 40% by weight through a sieve with a nominal mesh aperture of 250 μm.

3. Moderately Fine Powder

A powder all the particles of which pass through a sieve with a nominal mesh aperture of 355 μm and not more than 40% by weight through a sieve with a nominal mesh aperture of 180 μm.

4. Fine Powder

A powder all the particles of which pass through a sieve with nominal mesh aperture of 180 μm and not more than 40% by weight pass through a sieve with a nominal mesh aperture of 125 μm.

5. Very Fine Powder

A powder all the particles of which pass through a sieve with a nominal mesh aperture of 125 μm and not more than 40% by weight pass through a sieve with a nominal mesh aperture of 45 μm.

6. Microfine Powder

A powder of which not less than 90% by weight of the particles pass through a sieve with a nominal mesh aperture of 45 μm.

7. Superfine Powder

A powder of which not less than 90% by number of the particles are less than 10 μm in size.

When the fineness of the powder is described by means of a number, it is intended that all the particles of the powder shall pass through a sieve of which the nominal mesh aperture, in μm, is equal to that number.

Methods for Particle Size Determination

A number of methods are available for the determination of particle size of powders, including the following:

(a) Sieving

(b) Microscopy

(c) Sedimentation rate method

(d) Light energy diffraction or Light scattering method

(e) Laser holography

(f) Cascade impaction method

The above methods are used for the analysis of particle size and shape. Most of the commercially available particle size analyzers are automated and linked with computer for data processing, distribution analysis and printout.

On the basis of their intended use, powders may be grouped into following categories-

Powders for Oral Administration

Oral powders are preparations consisting of solid, loose, dry particles of varying degrees of fineness. They contain one or more medicaments with or without auxiliary substances including, where specified, flavoring and coloring agents. However, addition of saccharin or its salts is not permitted in the preparations meant for paediatric use.

Powders for oral administration generally consist of powder dosage forms intended to be swallowed directly into mouth or with water or other suitable liquid. Oral powders may be single dose or multiple dose preparations. For single dose powders, each dose is enclosed in a separate container, e.g., a sachet, a paper packet or a vial. With multiple dose powders it may be necessary to provide a measuring device capable of delivering the quantity prescribed. These types of powders are consisting of non-potent substances in bulk form like antacids, laxatives, purgatives etc.

Powders for the preparation of oral liquids are intended for the preparation of solution or suspension for oral use. Such preparations are used for drugs like antibiotics which are unstable in aqueous form and can not be prepared as liquid dosage form. Such powders are generally meant to be used within a short period of time after reconstitution.

Effervescent oral powders generally consist of suitable quantities of organic acids like tartaric or citric acid along with carbonates or bicarbonates that react rapidly in presence of water to release carbon dioxide. The ingredients of effervescent powders should be incorporated under the condition of controlled moisture to prevent the interactions between the ingredients and consequent loss of effervescences during manufacture. Effervescent oral powders are packed either in single dose or multi dose containers and are meant to be dissolved or dispersed in water before administration. The acidic and basic ingredients can also be dispensed separately with appropriate directions for use to the patients.

Standards for Oral Powders

(A) Uniformity of Content

Unless otherwise specified, oral powders presented in single dose containers that contain less than 10 mg of active ingredient per dose or that contain less than 10% w/w of active ingredient comply with this test. For oral powders containing more than one active ingredient carry out the test for each active ingredient that corresponds to the above conditions. For this test, empty each container as completely as possible and carry out the test on the individual contents of active ingredients.

The test for "uniformity of content" should be carried out only after the content of active ingredient(s) in a pooled sample of the preparation has been shown to be within the accepted limits of the stated content. Determine the content of active ingredient(s) of each of 10 containers taken at random using the method given in the monograph or by any other suitable analytical method of equivalent accuracy and precision. The preparation complies with the test if the individual values thus obtained are all between 85% to 115% of the average value.

The preparation fails to comply with the test if more than one individual value is outside the limits 85% to 115% of the average value or if any one individual value is outside the limits 75% to 125% of the average value. If one individual value is outside the limits 85% to 115 % but within the limits 75% to 125% of the average value, repeat the test using another 20 containers taken at random. The preparation complies with the test if in the total sample of 30 containers not more than 3 individual values are outside the limits 85% to 115% and not more than one is outside the limits 75% to 125% of the average value.

Note: The test for uniformity of content is not applicable to preparations containing multivitamins and trace elements.

(B)   Uniformity of Weight

Unless otherwise specified, oral powders presented in single dose containers comply with the test for contents of packaged dosage forms. This test and specifications apply to oral dosage forms and preparations that are packaged in containers in which the labeled net quantity is not more than 100 g. For this, select a sample of 10 filled containers and remove any labeling that might be altered in weight while removing the contents of the containers. Clean and dry the outer surfaces of the containers and weigh each container. Remove quantitatively the contents from each container. If necessary, cut open the container and wash each empty container with a suitable solvent, taking care to ensure that the closure and other parts of the container are retained. Dry and again weigh each empty container together with its parts which may have been removed. The difference between the two weights is the net weight of the contents of the container. The average net weight of the contents of the 10 containers is not less than the labeled amount and the net weight of the contents of any single containers is not less than 98% and not more than 109% of the labeled amount.

If this requirement is not met, count the number of the contents in each of 10 additional containers. The average number in the 20 containers is not less than the labeled amount, and the number is not more than 1 of the 20 containers is less than 98% or more than 102% or the labeled amount.

(C) Uniformity of Mass

Single-dose oral powders comply with the test for uniformity of mass of single-dose preparations. If the test for uniformity of content is prescribed for all the active substances, the test for uniformity of mass is not required. Oral powders supplied in multi-dose containers comply with the test of uniformity of mass of delivered doses from multi-dose containers.

Dusting Powders

Dusting powders are finely divided powders that are intended to be applied to the skin for therapeutic, prophylactic or lubricant purposes. In general, dusting powders should be passed through at least a 100 mesh sieve to assure freedom from dirt that could irritate traumatized areas. The essential characteristics of dusting powders include (a) homogeneity, (b) non-irritability, (c) free flowing, (d) good spreadability and covering capacity, (e) very fine particles size, (f) good adsorption and absorption capacity, and (g) capacity to protect the skin against roughness and irritation caused by friction, moisture or chemical irritants.

Dusting powders are of two types- Medical and Surgical Dusting powder. Medical dusting powders are used mainly for superficial skin conditions, whereas surgical dusting powders are used in body cavities and also on major wounds as a result of burns and umbilical cords of infants. Generally dusting powders should not be applied to the broken skin. Only sterile dusting powder should be applied to open wounds. Such preparation should be prepared using materials and methods designed to ensure sterility and to avoid the introduction of contaminants and the growth of microorganism. Surgical dusting powders must be sterilized before their use while medical dusting powders must be free from pathogenic microorganisms.

Dusting powders for lubricant purposes or superficial skin conditions need not be sterile but they should be free from pathogenic organism e.g., talc may be contaminated with spores of pathogen *Clostridium tetani* causing tetanus so it should be sterilized by dry heat prior to the incorporation into the product. Talc dusting powder is a sterile cutaneous powder containing starch and purified talc in which the talc is sterilized before incorporation with the starch, or the final product is subjected to a suitable terminal sterilization procedure.

Dusting powders are dispensed in sifter-top containers to facilitate dusting onto the skin. The powder must flow well from the container, so that it can be dusted over the affected area. The active ingredients must therefore be diluted with materials having good flow properties, e.g., purified talc or maize starch. Dusting powders are employed mainly as lubricants, protectives, astringents, absorbents, antiseptics, antipruritics and antiperspirants. Dusting powders should be stored in a dry place. The label of dusting powders should state (1) the date after which the dusting powder is not intended to be used, and (2) the conditions under which the dusting powder should be stored.

Dentifrices

Dentifrices or tooth powders are hygienic bulk powders which are used to clean teeth. They usually contain soap or detergent, mild abrasive and anticariogenic agent. Mild abrasion may be provided by incorporation of finely precipitated calcium carbonate or hydrous dibasic calcium phosphate. The abrasive action must be mild otherwise it damages the tooth enamel. The detergent action is given by the incorporation of soaps or other suitable surfactants. Flavoring, coloring and sweetening agents are also added with care. Essential oils are added to provide flavor and freshness to the mouth as well as antiseptic action. Uniform distribution of essential oils can be obtained by adsorbing them on abrasives.

Insufflations

Insufflations are finely divided powders intended for introduction into body cavities such as nose, ears, vagina with the help of insufflators. Insufflators are simple devices enabling blowing out of finely divided powders in a stream of gas by the application of mild pressure on the compression of bulb. Uniform dose delivery can not be regulated by insufflators. The electrostatic charges may be generated in the insufflators causing the particles to adhere to each other or to the wall of the insufflator. This drawback can be overcome by the use of aerosol packages. Generally insufflations are intended for local action but some of them can produce systemic effects also, e.g., intranasal insufflations. In insufflations the particle size must be very small and they should be absolutely free from irritant and sensitizing qualities.

Powders for Parenteral Administration

Powders for parenteral administration are sterile, solid fine particles including lyophilized materials packed in their final containers and which, when shaken with the prescribed volume of appropriate sterile liquid, rapidly form clear, practically particle free solutions or uniform suspensions. Such practice is applied for the drugs, which are unstable in the presence of water and can not be formulated in the form of a liquid injection e.g., antibiotics.

Methods of Preparation

During the manufacturing of oral powders, measures are taken to ensure a suitable particle size with regard to the intended use. In the manufacture, packaging, storage and distribution of oral powders, suitable means are taken to ensure their microbial quality.

Generally on laboratory scale, powders can be prepared with the help of mortar and pestle.

Therapeutic Uses

The powders are therapeutically used on the basis of the active constituents and type of powder. For example, oral rehydration salts are used for the prevention and treatment of dehydration. Dusting powders are used mainly as lubricants, protectives, absorbents, antiseptics, antipruritics and antiperspirants.

Dose

The dose of powders is as directed by physician.

Storage Conditions

Powders should be stored in tightly-closed containers. If the preparation contains volatile ingredients, or the contents have to be protected, store in an airtight container.

Specific Labeling Requirement

For single dose containers the label should state the name and quantity of active ingredient per container; and for multi-dose containers, the name and quantity of active ingredient in a suitable amount by weight. The label also states (1) the name and proportions of any antimicrobial preservative, (2) the directions for use of the oral powder, (3) the date after which the oral powder is not intended to be used, and (4) the conditions under which the oral powder should be stored. The label of dusting powders should state 'FOR EXTERNAL USE ONLY'.

Contraindication

The dusting powders should not be applied to the broken skin.

Examples of Some Powders

1. Oral Rehydration Salts IP; BP

Oral Rehydration Salts (ORS) are dry, homogeneously mixed oral powders containing cithcr anhydrous dcxtrosc or dcxtrosc monohydrate, sodium chloride, potassium chloride and either sodium citrate or sodium bicarbonate. After being dissolved in the requisite volume of water they are intended for the prevention and treatment of dehydration due to diarrhea, including maintenance therapy. They are odorless, white to creamy-white, amorphous or crystalline powder.

As the stability of oral rehydration salts containing sodium bicarbonate under tropical conditions is very poor, formulations containing sodium bicarbonate are less suitable; sodium bicarbonate may be packaged separately in such cases to improve storage stability. They may contain suitable flavoring agents and, where necessary, suitable flow agents in the minimum quantity required to achieve a satisfactory product but may not contain artificial sweetening agents like mono- and/or polysaccharides. If saccharin/saccharin sodium or aspartame is used in preparations meant for paediatric use, the concentration of saccharin should be such that its daily intake is not more than 5 mg/kg of body weight and that of aspartame should be such that its daily intake is not more than 40 mg/kg of body weight.

Oral Rehydration Salts-A, is commonly used in India for treatment of non-choleraic diarrhea while Diarrheal Diseases Control Programme of the World Health Organization (WHO) and the United Nations Children Fund (UNICEF) recommend the Oral Rehydration Salts-Citrate. The compositions of the two formulations as described by IP (1996) and WHO in terms of the amount, in g, to be dissolved in sufficient water to produce 1000 ml, are given below:

Ingredients	Formula (g/L)	
	ORS-A (IP)	ORS-Citrate (WHO)
Sodium chloride	1.25	3.5
Potassium chloride	1.5	1.5
Sodium citrate	2.9	2.9
Anhydrous dextrose **or** Dextrose monohydrate	27.0 29.7	20.0 22.0

A formulation of reduced osmolarity recommended by IP, 2007 is given below:

Ingredients	Quantity Required
Sodium chloride	2.6
Potassium chloride	1.5
Sodium citrate	2.9
Dextrose (anhydrous) **or** Dextrose monohydrate	13.5 14.85

The molar concentrations of ions in terms of mmol/L are- Sodium-75, Potassium-20, Chloride-65, Citrate-10 and Dextrose-75. The total osmolar concentration of the solution in terms of mOsmol/L is 245.

Composition	Method of Preparation
Each sachet contains, Sodium chloride- 2.6 g Potassium chloride- 1.5 g Sodium citrate- 2.9 g Anhydrous dextrose- 13.5 g	Finely powder the ingredients mentioned in the formula separately, using mortar and pestle. Then weigh accurately the required quantity of each ingredient and blend them by geometric dilution in ascending order of weights.

Label

ORS POWDER IP		
Composition: Each sachet contains, Sodium chloride- 2.6 g Potassium chloride- 1.5 g Sodium citrate- 2.9 g Anhydrous dextrose- 13.5 g *(The composition should be dissolved in 1 L water)* **Dose:** As directed by physician **Storage:** Store in air tight sachet in a dry and cool place.	**YAPHA-ORS** (Powders) **Oral Rehydration Salts** (Used for non-choleraic diarrhea and rehydration) **NOT FOR INJECTION** *(Solution prepared from the ORS powder that remains unused for 24 hours after preparation should be discarded)*	**Mfg. Lic. No.-**6H/2010 **Batch No.-** NM 0780 **Mfg. Date-** July 2011 **Exp. Date-** June 2012 **M.R.P.-** Rs. 15.00 (Inclusive of all taxes) **Mfd. By:** YAVI PHARMA KANPUR ROAD, LUCKNOW UP- 226001

2. Hexachlorophene Dusting Powder BPC

It is a cutaneous powder. The label of zinc and hexachlorophene dusting powder states that the preparation should not be applied to infants or to large areas of skin except in accordance with medical advice. It is a disinfectant powder with bacteriostatic activity against *Staphylococcus aureus* and used to the umbilicus of babies.

Composition	Method of Preparation
Hexachlorophane- 3 g Zinc oxide- 30 g Maize starch- 967 g	Triturate the required quantity of hexachlorophane and zinc oxide with maize starch then pass through a sieve of suitable mesh size and mix.

Label

HEXACHLOROPHENE DUSTING POWDER BPC (50 g)		
Composition: Each 50 g contains, Hexachlorophane- 0.15 g Zinc oxide- 1.5 g Maize Starch q.s.- 50 g **Storage:** Store in a well-closed container in cool place.	**HEXACHLOR** (Dusting Powder) (Used as disinfectant powder) **FOR EXTERNAL USE ONLY**	**Mfg. Lic. No.-** 3G/2010 **Batch No.-** BN 034 **Mfg. Date-** Mar. 2011 **Exp. Date-** Feb. 2012 **M.R.P.-** Rs. 27.00 (Inclusive of all taxes) **Mfd. By:** YAVI PHARMA KANPUR ROAD, LUCKNOW UP- 226001

3. Talc Dusting Powder BP

It is a sterile cutaneous powder of suitable fineness. Talc is a powdered, selected, natural, hydrated magnesium silicate. It may contain variable amounts of associated minerals among which chlorites (hydrated aluminum and magnesium silicate), magnesite (magnesium carbonate), calcite (calcium carbonate), and dolomite (calcium and magnesium carbonate) are predominant.

Composition	Method of Preparation
Starch- 10 g Purified talc q.s.-100 g	Triturate the required quantity of starch with the purified talc and passed through a sieve of suitable mesh size (250 µm). Either the purified talc is sterilized before use or the final product is subjected to a suitable sterilization procedure. *Note-Tapioca Starch may be used in place of maize starch, potato starch, rice starch or wheat starch.*

Label

<table>
<tr><td colspan="3" align="center">TALC DUSTING POWDER BP
(50 g)</td></tr>
<tr>
<td>Composition:
Each 50 g contains,
Starch- 5 g
Purified talc q.s.- 50 g

Storage: Store in a well-closed container in cool place.</td>
<td align="center">TALCDUST
(Dusting Powder)
(Used as absorbent)

FOR EXTERNAL USE ONLY</td>
<td>Mfg. Lic. No.- 5M/2010
Batch No.- KJ 0110
Mfg. Date- Mar. 2011
Exp. Date- Feb. 2012
M.R.P.- Rs. 22.00
(Inclusive of all taxes)
Mfd. By: YAVI PHARMA
KANPUR   ROAD, LUCKNOW
UP- 226001</td>
</tr>
</table>

4. Compound Clioquinol Topical Powder

Compound clioquinol topical powder contains not less than 22.5% and not more than 27.5% of clioquinol.

Composition	Method of Preparation
Clioquinol- 250 g Lactic acid- 25 g Zinc stearate- 200 g Lactose q.s. to-1000 g	Mix the required quantity of lactic acid with lactose then add the clioquinol and zinc stearate and mix them properly.

Label

COMPOUND CLIOQUINOL TOPICAL POWDER		
(50 g)		
Composition:		**Mfg. Lic. No.-** 5M/2010
Each 50 g contains,	**CLIOQUIN**	**Batch No.-** KJ 0110
Clioquinol- 12.5 g	(Topical Powder)	**Mfg. Date-** Mar., 2011
Lactic acid- 1.25 g		**Exp. Date-** Feb. 2012
Zinc stearate- 10 g		**M.R.P.-** Rs. 22.00
Lactose q.s. to- 50 g		(Inclusive of all taxes)
Storage: Store in a well-	**FOR EXTERNAL USE**	**Mfd. By:** YAVI PHARMA
closed light-resistant	**ONLY**	KANPUR ROAD, LUCKNOW
container in cool place.		UP- 226001

5. Methylbenzethonium Chloride Topical Powder

Methylbenzethonium chloride topical powder contains not less than 85% and not more than 115% of the labeled amount of methylbenzethonium chloride in a suitable powder base. Not less than 99% of this powder passes through a No. 200 sieve.

Composition	Method of Preparation
Methylbenzethonium chloride- 90 g	Mix the required quantity of methylbenzethonium chloride with suitable fine powder base, free from grittiness then passes through a
Powder base q.s. to-100 g	No. 200 sieve.

Label

METHYLBENZETHONIUM CHLORIDE TOPICAL POWDER		
(50 g)		
Composition:		**Mfg. Lic. No.-** 2G/2010
Each 50 g contains,	**METHBENZTOP**	**Batch No.-** JK 056
Methylbenzethonium	(Topical Powder)	**Mfg. Date-** June 2011
chloride- 45 g		**Exp. Date-** May 2012
Powder base q.s. to-50 g		**M.R.P.-** Rs. 28.00
		(Inclusive of all taxes)
	FOR EXTERNAL USE	
Storage: Store in a well-	**ONLY**	**Mfd. By:** YAVI PHARMA KANPUR
closed light-resistant		ROAD, LUCKNOW UP- 226001
container in cool place.		

6. Sodium Picosulphate Oral Powder BP

Sodium Picosulphate Oral Powder BP contains sodium picosuphate, light magnesium oxide and anhydrous citric acid. The content of sodium picosuphate, light magnesium oxide and anhydrous citric acid is 90% to 110% of the stated amount. The label of Sodium Picosuphate Oral Powder BP should state (1) the total weights of the constituents of sachet in grams (2) that heat is evolved when the contents of the sachet are added to water.

Composition	Method of Preparation
Sodium picosuphate- 0.1 g Light magnesium oxide- 3.5 g Anhydrous citric acid- 12 g	Mix the required quantity of powdered sodium picosuphate and light magnesium oxide with anhydrous citric acid.

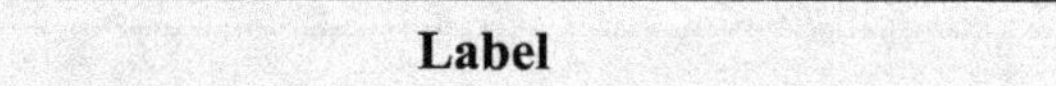

Label

<table>
<tr><td colspan="3" align="center">SODIUM PICOSUPHATE ORAL POWDER BP
(50 g)</td></tr>
<tr>
<td>Composition:
Each 50 g contains,
Sodium picosuphate- 0.3 g
Light magnesium oxide- 10.5 g
Anhydrous citric acid q.s.- 50 g
Dose: As directed by physician
Storage: Store in a well-closed light-resistant container in cool place.</td>
<td align="center">PICOSUL
(Powder)
(Used as laxative)

PROTECT FROM SUN LIGHT</td>
<td>Mfg. Lic. No.- 2F/2010
Batch No.- BN 0110
Mfg. Date- Sep. 2011
Exp. Date- Aug. 2012
M.R.P.- Rs. 25.00
(Inclusive of all taxes)
Mfd. By: YAVI PHARMA KANPUR ROAD, LUCKNOW UP- 226001</td>
</tr>
</table>

7. Compound Rhubarb Powder (Gregory's Powder) BPC

Composition	Method of Preparation
Rhubarb (powdered form)- 250 g Ginger (powdered form)- 100 g Light magnesium carbonate- 325 g Heavy magnesium carbonate- 325 g	Weigh the required quantities of ingredients and powder them separately. Mix all the ingredients in ascending order of their weights and transfer the powder in a wide mouthed bottle.

Label

COMPOUND RHUBARB POWDER (GREGORY'S POWDER) BPC (50 g)		
Composition: Each 50 g contains, Rhubarb (powdered)- 12.5 g Ginger (powdered)- 5 g Light magnesium carbonate- 16.25 g Heavy magnesium carbonate- 16.25 g **Dose:** 0.5 to 5 g two times a day. **Storage:** Store in a well-closed container in cool place.	**COMRHUBA** (Powders) (Used as Purgative) **PROTECT FROM SUN LIGHT**	**Mfg. Lic. No.-** 2L/2010 **Batch No.-** CV 036 **Mfg. Date-** Nov. 2011 **Exp. Date-** Oct. 2012 **M.R.P.-** Rs. 24.00 (Inclusive of all taxes) **Mfd. By:** YAVI PHARMA KANPUR ROAD, LUCKNOW UP- 226001

Marketed Preparations

Active Ingredient(s)	Marketed preparation (Manufacturer)
Glucosamine	**FLEXTRA** (ELDER H. CARE), **BIG JOINT** (BESTOCHEM)
Sodium aminosalicylate	**Q-PAS** (LUPIN)
Isabgol	**BOWLAX** (BIOSTRASS), **CREMAFFIN-FS** (ABBOTT), **FEEL GOOD** (ZEE LAB), **FIBRIL** (LUPIN), **FYBOGEL** (NICHOLAS PIRAMAL), **ISADIET** (MARC LAB)
Clotrimazole	**ABZORB** (CROSLAND), **CANDID** (GLENMARK), **CEZEL** (OREVA DERMACARE), **CLOBEN DUSTING POWDER** (INDOCO), **D-ZORB** (D.M. CARE BIOTECH), **MYCODERM-C** (FDC), **SURFAZ** (FRANCO-INDIAN), **TOLODERM** (DR. DERMA)
Silver sulphadiazine	**SILVEREX** (CROSLANDS)
Electrolytes	**AGITRAL** (AGRAWAL PHARMA), **BESTOLYTE** (BESTOCHEM), **ELECTRAL** (FDC), **LECYTE** (ALBERT DAVID), **PEDIALYTE** (PFIZER), **ORFIZ** (NOVARTIS), **RECOLYTE** (ALWIN WILLCURE)
Proteins	**ELNUTRIN** C (ELDER), **AVIPRO** (ENDOCARD INDIA), **CADPRO** (ZYDUS), **HALPRO-DHA** (HALLMARK), **KOMPRO** (PLUS INDIA), **MAGVIT PRO** (MAGNUS BIOTECH), **PRD** (UNITED LIFECARE), **PROVITAX** (INNOVA)

EXERCISE - 11

Object

To prepare and submit 50 g ORS Powder IP.

Theory

Pharmaceutical powders are dosage forms of medicament, in which one or more drugs are dispensed in a finely divided state, with or without excipients. Powders are available in crystalline or amorphous form. Oral Rehydration Salts (ORS) are dry, homogeneously mixed powders containing dextrose, sodium chloride, potassium chloride and either sodium bicarbonate or sodium citrate for use in oral rehydration therapy after being dissolved in requisite amount of water. As the stability of Oral Rehydration Salts containing sodium bicarbonate under tropical conditions is very poor, formulations containing sodium bicarbonate are less suitable; sodium bicarbonate may be packaged separately in such cases to improve storage stability. Oral Rehydration Salts may contain suitable flavoring agents and, where necessary, suitable flow agents in the minimum quantity required to achieve a satisfactory product but may not contain artificial sweetening agents like mono- or polysaccharides, saccharin or aspartame.

Formula

The composition should be dissolved in sufficient water to produce 1000 ml.

Ingredients	Quantity Required
Sodium chloride	1.25 g
Potassium chloride	1.5 g
Sodium citrate	2.9 g
Anhydrous dextrose **or**	27 g
Dextrose monohydrate	29.7 g

Apparatus

Mortar and pestle, spatula.

Procedure

Finely powder the ingredients mentioned in the formula separately, using mortar and pestle. Then weigh accurately the required quantity of each ingredient and blend them by geometric dilution in ascending order of weights. Transfer it in suitable container and close it tightly.

Category

Replacement solution for diarrheal rehydration.

Dose

The composition should be dissolved in 1000 ml of water and solution should be taken as directed by physician within 24 hours after the preparation of solution.

Therapeutic Use

ORS Powder IP is commonly used for treatment of non-choleraic diarrhea to maintain the homeostasis. After being dissolved in the requisite volume of water ORS Powder IP is intended for the prevention and treatment of dehydration due to diarrhea, including maintenance therapy.

Storage

ORS Powder IP should be protected from moisture so they should be stored in tightly-closed containers in a dry and cool place. Sachets, preferably made of aluminium foil, containing sufficient powder for a single dose or for a day's treatment are usually satisfactory to prevent ingress of moisture. Powders for use in hospitals may be presented in bulk containers containing sufficient quantity to produce a volume of solution appropriate to the daily requirements of the hospital concerned.

Label

The label of ORS Powder IP should state (1) the appropriate title, viz Oral Rehydration Salts-A or Oral Rehydration Salts-Citrate, (2) for sachets, the total weight, in gram of the constituents, (3) for bulk containers the weight in gram of the constituents in a stated quantity, in gram of the powder, (4) the total weight of the contents of the container, (5) the directions for use, (6) that any portion of the solution prepared from the oral powder that remains unused for 24 hours after preparation should be discarded, and (7) the storage conditions.

Specimen Label

The specimen label for ORS Powder IP is given as:

ORS POWDER IP		
Composition: Each sachet contains, Sodium Chloride- 1.25 g Potassium Chloride- 1.5 g Sodium Citrate- 2.9 g Anhydrous Dextrose- 27 g *(The composition should be dissolved in 1 L water)* **Dose:** As directed by physician **Storage:** Store in tightly-closed containers in a dry and cool place.	**YAVI ORS** (Powders) **Oral Rehydration Salts-A** (Used for non-choleraic diarrhea and rehydration) **NOT FOR INJECTION** *(Solution prepared from the ORS powder that remains unused for 24 hours after preparation should be discarded)*	**Mfg. Lic. No.-** 5C/2010 **Batch No.-** BK 0224 **Mfg. Date-** Feb. 2011 **Exp. Date-** Jan. 2012 **M.R.P.-** Rs. 15.00 (Inclusive of all taxes) **Mfd. By:** YAVI PHARMA KANPUR ROAD, LUCKNOW UP- 226001

EXERCISE - 12

Object

To prepare and submit 50 g Absorbable Dusting Powder USP/NF.

Theory

Dusting powders are bulk powders meant for external application to the skin for various purposes. Dusting powders should be homogeneous and in a very fine state of subdivision to enhance the effectiveness of the medicament and minimize the local irritation. In addition, dusting powders should have free flowability, easy spreadability, non irritability, non grittiness, good absorption and adsorption capacities and compatible with skin secretions.

Absorbable dusting powder USP/NF is an absorbable powder prepared by processing corn starch and intended for use as a lubricant for surgical gloves. It contains not more than 2% of magnesium oxide.

Formula

Ingredients	Quantity Required
Magnesium oxide	2 g
Corn starch	98 g

Apparatus

Mortar and pestle, spatula.

Procedure

Finely powder the ingredients mentioned in the formula separately, using mortar and pestle. Then weigh accurately the required quantity of each ingredient and blend them by geometric dilution in ascending order of weights. Transfer it in suitable container and close it tightly.

Category

Dusting powder.

Dose

As directed by physician.

Therapeutic Use

Lubricant for surgical gloves.

Storage

Absorbable dusting powder USP/NF should be preserved in well closed containers. It may be preserved in sealed paper packets.

Label

The label should have the cautions 'FOR EXTERNAL USE ONLY', 'STORE IN A DRY PLACE', 'NOT FOR INJECTION'.

Caution

Absorbable dusting powder USP/NF should not be applied on open wounds and broken skin.

Specimen Label

The specimen label for Absorbable Dusting Powder USP/NF is given as:

<table>
<tr><td colspan="3" align="center">ABSORBABLE DUSTING POWDER USP/NF
(50 g)</td></tr>
<tr>
<td valign="top">Composition:
Each 50 g contains,
Magnesium oxide-1g
Corn starch- 49 g
Dose: As directed by physician
Storage: Store in well closed
container in cool and dry place.</td>
<td valign="top" align="center">YAVISORB
(Dusting powder)
(Used as a lubricant for surgical gloves)

FOR EXTERNAL USE ONLY
NOT FOR INJECTION
(It should not be applied on open
wounds and broken skin)</td>
<td valign="top">Mfg. Lic. No.- 2C/2010
Batch No.- YM 0135
Mfg. Date- Nov. 2011
Exp. Date- Oct. 2012
M.R.P.- Rs. 35.00
(Inclusive of all taxes)
Mfd. By: YAVI
PHARMA KANPUR
ROAD, LUCKNOW
UP- 226001</td>
</tr>
</table>

CHAPTER 7

LOTIONS

A lotion is a low- to medium-viscous, topical preparation intended for application to unbroken skin. Pharmaceutically lotions are suspensions of solid materials in aqueous vehicle, although certain emulsions and true solutions have also been designated as lotions because of either their appearance or applications. Lotions may be preferred over semisolid preparations because of their non-greasy nature and improved spreadability over large area of skin. Lotions differ from creams as creams are inappropriate for application to regions of hairy skin such as the scalp, while a lotion is less viscous and may be readily applied to these areas (many medicated shampoos are the examples of lotions). Historically, lotions also had an advantage in that they may be spread thinly compared to a cream and may economically cover a large area of skin.

Lotions are usually applied to external skin with bare hands, a clean cloth, cotton wool or gauze. Many lotions, especially Hand Creams and Face Cream are formulated not as a medicine delivery system, but simply to smooth and soften the skin. These are particularly popular with the aging and aged demographic groups, and in the case of face usage, can also be classified as a cosmetic in many cases. The key components of a skin care lotion are the aqueous and oily phases, an emulgent to prevent separation of these two phases, and, if used, a medicament. A wide variety of other ingredients such as fragrances, glycerol, dyes, preservatives and stabilizing agents are generally added to lotions.

Lotions are designed to be applied to the unbroken skin without friction. They may contain humectants; so that moisture is retained on surface of the skin after its application. Lotions may also contain alcohol which evaporates rapidly, imparting a cooling effect and leaving the skin dry.

Methods of Preparation

Lotions may be prepared by triturating the ingredients to make a smooth paste and then diluting it carefully with the remaining liquid phase with trituration to make up the desired volume. High speed mixers or colloidal mills produce better dispersions therefore are used in a preparation of larger quantities of lotion. Calamine Lotion USP is the classical example of this type of preparation. Although most of the lotions are prepared by trituration, some lotions like White Lotion NF are prepared by chemical interaction in the liquid.

Therapeutic Uses

Lotions are used for the protective or therapeutic value of their ingredients e.g., Calamine Lotion USP is used as an astringent and protective against sun burn and other itching conditions. Benzyl Benzoate Lotion USP is used in the treatment of scabies and as a pediculicide. Lotions can also be used for the delivery of medications such as antibiotics, antiseptics, antifungal, corticosteroids, anti-acne agents, soothing, smoothing, moisturizing or protective agents (such as calamine) to the skin.

Lead lotions are empirical treatments for sprains and bruises. Other lotions contain medicaments for treating skin conditions e.g., copper with zinc sulphates are used for impetigo, zinc with salicylic acid for ulcers, salicylic acid for dandruff, salicylic acid with mercuric chloride for follicular infections. Copper and zinc sulphates are astringents while salicylic acid is keratolytic, bacteriostatic and fungicidal.

Dose

Lotions are applied topically.

Storage Conditions

The lotions should be stored in a well filled, well-closed air tight container in a cool place. Do not freeze.

Specific Labeling Requirement

The label should state the names and concentrations of the active ingredients in the preparation. Since lotions are topical preparations so its container should be labeled 'FOR EXTERNAL USE ONLY'. If the lotion is suspension type, then the container must be labeled 'SHAKE WELL BEFORE USE'.

The label should also state the date after which the lotion is not intended to be used, the conditions under which the lotion should be stored, the directions for using the lotion and any special precautions associated with the use of the lotion.

Since Salicylic acid Lotion and Salicylic acid with Mercuric chloride Lotion contain 95% alcohol and acetone with 95% alcohol, respectively so these preparations must be labeled to indicate their high inflammability.

Examples of Some Lotions

1. Calamine Lotion IP; BP; USP

Calamine lotion is a topic treatment that combines zinc oxide and iron (III) oxide to produce a lotion, which is utilized to help mitigate irritants associated contact dermatitis. Calamine lotion often appears as pink in color and has a thick, creamy texture in many cases. It is sold primarily as a generic and is available over the counter in many countries. Chemically calamine is a mixture of zinc oxide (ZnO) with about 0.5% iron oxide (Fe_2O_3). Calamine is the main ingredient in calamine lotion.

Calamine lotion is used as an antipruritic (anti-itching agent) to treat mild pruritic conditions such as sunburn, eczema, rashes, insect bites and stings.

It is also used as a mild antiseptic to prevent infections that can be caused by scratching the affected area and an astringent to dry weeping or oozing blisters. Calamine lotion can also be used to treat acne, though it may not be as proficient in treating the problem as some of the other topical treatments available. However, use of the lotion may provide some immediately benefits, such as lessening the irritation and making the blemishes blend in with the skin a little better.

Calamine lotion is thought to be able to help soothe and protect the skin when it becomes irritated so it acts as soothing, smoothing and moisturizing agent. It is often used in treating symptoms associated with poison ivy infection and chicken pox.

When using calamine lotion around the face, care should be taken to avoid the eyes and other mucous membranes. Calamine lotion has a tendency to dry out the skin and if it contacts these areas it can become an irritant itself.

Calamine lotion is usually applied on a daily basis, often twice or more daily as conditions demand. It is rare to have any serious, negative side effects resulting from the use of calamine lotion.

Calamine Lotion IP	Calamine Lotion BP	Calamine Lotion USP
Composition: Calamine- 150 g Zinc oxide- 50 g Bentonite- 30 g Sodium citrate- 5 g Liquefied phenol- 5 ml Glycerin- 50 ml Purified water (freshly boiled and cooled) q.s.- 1000 ml **Method of preparation:** Triturate the required quantity of	Calamine Lotion BP has similarity to that of Calamine Lotion IP in the form of ingredients, their amounts and also in method of preparation.	**Composition:** Calamine- 80 g Zinc oxide- 80 g Glycerin- 20 ml Bentonite magma- 250 ml Calcium hydroxide q.s.- 1000 ml **Method of preparation:** Dilute the bentonite magma with an equal volume of calcium hydroxide solution. Mix the required quantity of powdered

Table *Contd...*

<table>
<tr><td valign="top">

calamine, zinc oxide and bentonite with a solution of the sodium citrate in about 700 ml of purified water and add the liquefied phenol, glycerin and sufficient purified water to produce 1000 ml.

Note- Microbial limit of Calamine Lotion IP is described as "1 g should be free from *Staphylococcus aureus* and 10 g should be free from *Pseudomonas aeruginosa"*.

</td><td></td><td valign="top">

ingredients intimately with the glycerin and about 100 ml of the diluted magma, triturating until a smooth, uniform paste is formed. Gradually incorporate the remainder of the diluted magma. Finally add enough calcium hydroxide solution to make 1000 ml and shake well.

If a more viscous consistency is desired, the quantity of bentonite magma may be increased but not more than 400 ml.

Note - Calamine Lotion USP should meet the requirements of the tests for absence of *Staphylococcus aureus* and *Pseudomonas aeruginosa.*

</td></tr>
</table>

Label

<table>
<tr><td colspan="3" align="center">

CALAMINE LOTION USP

(50 ml)

</td></tr>
<tr><td valign="top">

Composition:

Each 50 ml contains,

Calamine- 80 g

Zinc oxide- 80 g

Glycerin- 20 ml

Bentonite magma- 250 ml

Calcium hydroxide q.s.- 1000 ml

Dose: As directed by physician

Storage: Store in airtight container.

</td><td valign="top" align="center">

CALMIN-LOTION

(Lotion)

(Used as antipruritic and mild antiseptic)

SHAKE WELL BEFORE USE

FOR EXTERNAL USE ONLY

</td><td valign="top">

Mfg. Lic. No.- 4H/2010

Batch No.- BN 0115

Mfg. Date- Feb. 2011

Exp. Date- Jan. 2012

M.R.P.- Rs. 20.00

(Inclusive of all taxes)

Mfd. By: YAVI PHARMA KANPUR ROAD, LUCKNOW UP- 226001

</td></tr>
</table>

2. Benzyl Benzoate Lotion USP

It contains not less than 26% and not more than 30% w/w of benzyl benzoate ($C_{14}H_{12}O_2$). It has pH 8.5 to 9.2.

Composition	Method of Preparation
Benzyl benzoate- 250 ml Triethanolamine- 5 g Oleic acid- 20 g Purified water q.s.- 1000 ml	Mix the required quantity of triethanolamine with oleic acid, add benzyl benzoate and mix. Transfer the mixture to a suitable container of about 2000 ml capacity, add 250 ml purified water and shake the mixture thoroughly. Finally add the remaining purified water to make up the volume 1000 ml and again shake thoroughly.

Label

<table>
<tr><td colspan="3" align="center">BENZYL BENZOATE LOTION USP
(50 ml)</td></tr>
<tr>
<td>Composition:
Each 50 ml contains,
Benzyl benzoate- 12.5 ml
Triethanolamine- 0.25 g
Oleic acid- 1 g
Purified water q.s.- 50 ml
Dose: As directed by physician
Storage: Store in tight container.</td>
<td align="center">BENZO-LOTION
(Lotion)
(Used for the treatment of scabies and as pediculicide)

SHAKE WELL BEFORE USE FOR EXTERNAL USE ONLY</td>
<td>Mfg. Lic. No.- 5M/2010
Batch No.- KJ 0110
Mfg. Date- Mar. 2011
Exp. Date- Feb. 2012
M.R.P.- Rs. 22.00
(Inclusive of all taxes)
Mfd. By: YAVI PHARMA KANPUR ROAD, LUCKNOW UP- 226001</td>
</tr>
</table>

3. Benzoyl Peroxide Lotion BP

Benzoyl Peroxide Lotion BP is a cutaneous suspension. It contains anhydrous benzoyl peroxide in a suitable non-greasy vehicle. The content of anhydrous benzoyl peroxide ($C_{14}H_{10}O_4$) in the lotion is 90 to 110% of the stated amount. In the label of Benzoyl Peroxide Lotion BP the quantity of active ingredient is stated in terms of the equivalent amount of anhydrous benzoyl peroxide.

Composition	Method of Preparation
Benzoyl Peroxide- 5 g Purified water q.s.- 100 ml	Mix the required quantity of benzoyl peroxide in 100 ml of purified water and shake the mixture thoroughly.

Label

<table>
<tr><td colspan="3" align="center">BENZOYL PEROXIDE LOTION BP
(50 ml)</td></tr>
<tr>
<td>Composition:
Each 50 ml contains,
Benzoyl peroxide- 2.5 g
Purified water q.s.- 50 ml
Dose: As directed by physician
Storage: Store in tight container.</td>
<td align="center">BENPER-LOTION
(Lotion)
(Used for acne)

SHAKE WELL BEFORE USE
FOR EXTERNAL USE ONLY</td>
<td>Mfg. Lic. No.- 2D/2010
Batch No.- CN 078
Mfg. Date- Sep. 2011
Exp. Date- Aug. 2012
M.R.P.- Rs. 27.00
(Inclusive of all taxes)
Mfd. By: YAVI PHARMA
KANPUR ROAD,
LUCKNOW UP- 226001</td>
</tr>
</table>

4. Sodium Bicarbonate Eye Lotion BP

Sodium Bicarbonate Eye Lotion BP is a sterile aqueous solution of sodium bicarbonate. It is an extemporaneous preparation. For the preparation of Sodium Bicarbonate Eye Lotion BP, dissolve the required quantity of sodium bicarbonate in sufficient purified water, clarify it by filtration then transfer the filtered solution into the final container, close the container so as to exclude microorganisms and sterilize by autoclaving.

The eye lotion complies with the requirements as per the norm of sterile preparations as well as ophthalmic formulations. In this lotion the content of sodium bicarbonate ($NaHCO_3$) is 90-110% of the stated amount.

Sodium Bicarbonate Eye Lotion BP should be supplied in suitable container with a nominal volume of not more than 1 L. Containers that have previously been subjected to heating in an autoclave should not be reused to keep eye lotion. The label of Sodium Bicarbonate Eye Lotion BP should state that the eye lotion not used within 24 hours of opening the container should be discarded. When Sodium Bicarbonate Eye Lotion BP is prescribed and no strength being stated, a lotion containing 2% w/v of sodium bicarbonate shall be dispensed.

Composition	Method of preparation
Sodium Bicarbonate- 2 g Purified water q.s.- 100 ml	Mix the required quantity of sodium bicarbonate in 100 ml of purified water and shake the solution thoroughly.

Label

<table>
<tr><td colspan="3" align="center">SODIUM BICARBONATE EYE LOTION BP
(50 ml)</td></tr>
<tr>
<td>Composition:
Each 50 ml contains,
Sodium Bicarbonate- 1 g
purified water q.s.- 50 ml
Dose: As directed by physician
Storage: Store in tight container.</td>
<td align="center">SOBICA-LOTION
(Lotion)
(Used as eye lubricant)

SHAKE WELL BEFORE USE
FOR EXTERNAL USE ONLY</td>
<td>Mfg. Lic. No.- 2D/2010
Batch No.- CN 078
Mfg. Date- Sep. 2011
Exp. Date- Aug. 2012
M.R.P.- Rs. 27.00
(Inclusive of all taxes)
Mfd. By: YAVI PHARMA KANPUR ROAD, LUCKNOW UP- 226001</td>
</tr>
</table>

5. White Lotion NF

White Lotion NF is a suspension prepared by chemical reaction between zinc sulphate and sulphurated potash. Sulphurated potash is a mixture of potassium polysulphites and potassium thiosulphate.

Composition	Method of Preparation	Caution
Zinc sulphate- 40 g Sulphurated potash- 40 g Purified water q.s.- 1000 ml	Dissolve the required quantity of zinc sulphate and sulphurated potash separately each in 450 ml of purified water and filter each solution. Add sulphurated potash solution slowly to the zinc sulphate solution with constant stirring. A finely divided precipitate of zinc sulphide is obtained that is diffusible in nature. Then add remaining amount of purified water to make up the volume 1000 ml and mix.	Zinc sulphate solution should not be added to the solution of sulphurated potash because it causes the formation of basic zinc salts and zinc hydroxide rather than zinc sulphide.

Label

<table>
<tr><td colspan="3" align="center">WHITE LOTION NF
(50 ml)</td></tr>
<tr>
<td>Composition:
Each 50 ml contains,
Zinc sulphate- 40 g
Sulphurated potash- 40 g
Purified water q.s.- 1000 ml
Dose: As directed by physician
Storage: Store in tight container.</td>
<td align="center">WHITO-LOTION
(Lotion)
(Used as astringent and protectant in acne)

SHAKE WELL BEFORE USE
FOR EXTERNAL USE ONLY</td>
<td>Mfg. Lic. No.- 5C/2010
Batch No.- AL 025
Mfg. Date- Nov. 2011
Exp. Date- Oct. 2012
M.R.P.- Rs. 21.00
(Inclusive of all taxes)
Mfd. By: YAVI PHARMA KANPUR ROAD, LUCKNOW UP- 226001</td>
</tr>
</table>

6. Amphotericin-B Lotion USP

Amphotericin-B is a mixture of antifungal polyenes produced by the growth of certain strains of *Streptomyces nodosus*. Amphotericin-B is a yellow or orange powder, which is practically insoluble in water and ethyl alcohol. It is slightly soluble in dimethylformamide but soluble in dimethyl sulphoxide and in propylene glycol. It is sensitive to light in dilute solutions and is inactivated at low pH values.

Amphotericin-B Lotion USP contains not less than 90% and not more than 125% of the labeled amount of Amphotericin-B. It has pH between 5 to 7. Amphotericin-B has a potency of not less than 750 µg of Amphotericin-B per mg calculated on the dried basis.

Composition	Method of Preparation
Amphotericin-B- 3 g Aqueous lotion vehicle q.s.- 100 ml	Weigh the required quantity of Amphotericin-B, mix with aqueous lotion vehicle and make the volume to 100 ml.

Label

<table>
<tr><td colspan="3" align="center">AMPHOTERICIN-B LOTION USP
(50 ml)</td></tr>
<tr>
<td>Composition:
Each 50 ml contains,
Amphotericin-B- 1.5 g
Aqueous lotion vehicle q.s.- 50 ml
Dose: As directed by physician
Storage: Store in tight, light-resistant container in a cold place (a temperature of 2°C-8°C).</td>
<td>AMPHO-LOTION
(Lotion)
(Used as antifungal agent)

SHAKE WELL BEFORE USE

FOR EXTERNAL USE ONLY</td>
<td>Mfg. Lic. No.- 3M/2010
Batch No.- HJ 124
Mfg. Date- Mar. 2011
Exp. Date- Feb. 2012
M.R.P.- Rs. 35.00
(Inclusive of all taxes)
Mfd. By: YAVI PHARMA KANPUR ROAD, LUCKNOW UP- 226001</td>
</tr>
</table>

Marketed preparations

Active Ingredient(s)	Marketed preparation (Manufacturer)
Fluconazole	**ZOCON** (FDC)
Dimethyl phthalate	**MYLOL** (ABBOTT)
Peppermint	**SANSUR LOTION** (GRACEWELL)
Clotrimazole	**CANDID** (GLENMARK), **CEZEL** (OREVA DERMACARE), **CLOBEN** (INDOCO), **MILAN MP** (MEFRO DERMACARE), **STATUM** (REXTAR)

Table *Contd...*

Active Ingredient(s)	Marketed preparation (Manufacturer)
Ketoconazole	**D-KETO** (D.M. CARE BIOTECH), **ZEE** (ZEE LAB), **K-CON** (UNITECH), **KETOCER** (AVENCER LABS), **KONAZ-CT** (TALENT INDIA)
Benzyl benzoate	**BENZYL BENZOATE APPLICATION** (AGRAWAL PHARMA)
Gamma benzene hexachloride	**AMEXIL** (LANARK), **BESTO-SCAB** (BESTOCHEM), **GAMMA BENZENE HEXACHLORIDE** (AGRAWAL PHARMA), **SCABOMA** (GLENMARK)
Gamma benzene hexachloride and Cetrimide	**GAMNIC-C** (SYNTONIC), **MAGSCAB** (MAGNUS BIOTECH), **SCABEX** (INDOCO), **SCABINE** (STADMED)
Beclomethasone	**BECARE** (CANBRO H. CARE)
Betamethasone	**BEZE LOTION** (ZEE LAB), **DIPROVATE** (CROSLANDS), **MONOVATE** (MEFRO DERMACARE), **ROVATE** (COSME H. CARE), **VALBET SCALP APPLICATION** (LUPIN)
Betamethasone and Salicylic acid	**SALTOPIC** (SYSTOPIC), **DIPSALIC** (FULFORD)
Clobetasol and Salicylic acid	**COVATE-S** (CANBRO H. CARE), **KLOSOL** (MEFRO DERMACARE), **STERIANATE** (SEGMENT CARE),**TOPISAL** (SYSTOPIC)
Miconazole	**ZOLE-F** (REXCEL RANBAXY)
Mmometasone	**CUTIZONE** (CROSLANDS), **FUROMATE** (SEGMENT CARE), **MMF** (OREVA DERMACARE), **STEROMOM** (ELDER)
Calamine	**CALADRYL** (PFIZER), **CALAWIN** (OREVA DERMACARE), **CALMIS** (AGRAWAL PHARMA), **CALOVERA** (AGRAWAL PHARMA), **LACTOCALAMINE** (PIRAMAL HEALTH CARE)

EXERCISE - 13

Object

To prepare and submit 50 ml Calamine Lotion IP.

Theory

Lotions are liquid or semi liquid preparations meant for external application to the skin without rubbing (friction). Calamine Lotion IP is a suspension containing indiffusible solids like calamine and zinc oxide. Calamine is a mixture of 98% zinc oxide with a small proportion of ferric oxide. Ferric oxide imparts a distinctive pink color to the zinc oxide for giving flesh like color to the lotion. Both calamine and zinc oxide are indiffusible in nature hence to make them diffusible uniformly in the vehicle, bentonite is used as a suspending agent. Bentonite is a natural colloidal hydrated aluminium silicate. Calamine Lotion IP also contains sodium citrate to prevent the lotion form being too viscous. It acts as a buffer and maintains the pH appropriate for skin preparations. Liquefied phenol acts as antipruritic. Glycerin acts as a hygroscopic agent and keeps the skin moist and produces soothening effect on the skin.

Microbial limit of Calamine Lotion IP is stated as "1 g should be free from *Staphylococcus aureus* and 10 g should be free from *Pseudomonas aeruginosa*".

Formula

Ingredients	Quantity Required
Calamine	150 g
Zinc oxide	50 g
Bentonite	30 g
Sodium citrate	5 g
Liquefied phenol	5 ml
Glycerin	50 ml
Purified water (freshly boiled and cooled) q.s. to	1000 ml

Apparatus

Glass beaker, measuring cylinder, mortar and pestle and volumetric pipette.

Procedure

Weigh the required quantity of calamine, zinc oxide and bentonite and mix them in mortar with pestle. Triturate it with a solution of weighed quantity of sodium citrate in about 700 ml. Add the required quantity of liquefied phenol and glycerin then mix well. To this mixture, add more of purified water (freshly boiled and cooled) to produce the required volume of 1000 ml. Mix thoroughly to get a uniform preparation.

Category

Protective lotion.

Dose

As directed by physician.

Therapeutic Use

Calamine Lotion IP is used as an antipruritic (anti-itching agent) to treat mild pruritic conditions such as sunburn, prickly heat, eczema, rashes, poison ivy, chicken pox, insect bites and stings. It is also used as a mild antiseptic to prevent infections that can be caused by scratching the affected area and an astringent to dry weeping or oozing blisters and acne abscesses. It also acts as soothing and moisturizing agent and gives protection from sunburn. It should be applied to the effected part without rubbing whenever necessary.

Storage

Calamine Lotion IP should be stored in well closed, narrow mouthed, fluted plastic bottle in cool place and close it tightly with plastic screw cap.

Label

'FOR EXTERNAL USE ONLY', 'SHAKE WELL BEFORE USE' and 'DO NOT FREEZE'.

Specimen Label

The specimen label for Calamine Lotion IP is given as:

<table>
<tr><td colspan="3" align="center">CALAMINE LOTION IP
(50 ml)</td></tr>
<tr><td>Composition:
Each 50 ml contains,
Calamine- 7.5 g
Zinc oxide- 2.5 g
Glycerin- 2.5 ml
Purified water q.s.- 50 ml
Dose: As directed by physician
Storage: Store in well closed, narrow mouthed, fluted plastic bottle in cool place.</td><td align="center">CALVI LOTION
(Lotion)

Protective Lotion
(Used as anti-itching agent and gives protection from sunburn)

FOR EXTERNAL USE ONLY
SHAKE WELL BEFORE USE
DO NOT FREEZE</td><td>Mfg. Lic. No.- 2V/2010
Batch No.- YM 0512
Mfg. Date- Mar. 2011
Exp. Date- Feb. 2012
M.R.P.- Rs. 35.00
(Inclusive of all taxes)
Mfd. By: YAVI PHARMA KANPUR ROAD, LUCKNOW UP- 226001</td></tr>
</table>

EXERCISE - 14

Object

To prepare and submit 50 ml Amino Benzoic Acid Lotion BP.

Theory

Lotions are liquid or semi liquid preparations meant for external application to the skin without friction. Lotion may be aqueous or alcoholic solutions or suspensions in aqueous medium. Amino benzoic acid lotion is a sunscreen lotion that absorbs or reflects some of the sun's ultraviolet (UV) radiation on the skin exposed to sunlight and thus helps protect against sunburn. The lotion protects lightened skin because light skin is more susceptible to sun damage than darker skin.

Sun Protection Factor (SPF)

The sun protection factor of a sunscreen is a laboratory measure of the effectiveness of sunscreen. The higher the SPF, the more protection a sunscreen offers against UV-B (the ultraviolet radiation that causes sunburn). The SPF is the amount of UV radiation required to cause sunburn on skin with the sunscreen on, relative to the amount required without the sunscreen. So, a lotion having SPF 50, will protect skin from burning until it has been exposed to 50 times the amount of solar energy that would normally cause it to burn.

Formula

Ingredients	Quantity Required
Amino benzoic acid	5 g
Glycerin	50 ml
Bentonite	10 g
Purified water q.s. to	100 ml

Apparatus

Glass beaker, measuring cylinder, mortar and pestle and volumetric pipette.

Procedure

Weigh the required quantity of ingredients and mix them in a mortar with pestle, triturate with glycerin and mix well, and add more of purified water (freshly boiled and cooled) to produce the required volume of 100 ml. Mix thoroughly to get a uniform preparation.

Category

Sun protective.

Dose

As directed by physician. Apply evenly and liberally to all exposed areas of the skin 30 minutes prior to exposure to the sun.

Therapeutic Use

It is used to prevent chapped dry skin and softens the texture of the skin. Amino benzoic acid Lotion provides natural protection with its UV absorption qualities. It prevents sunburn and protects skin from the harmful effects of the sun.

Storage

Amino benzoic acid Lotion BP should be stored in well closed, narrow mouthed, fluted plastic bottle in cool place, tightly closed with plastic screw cap. Preferable temperature of storage is between 15°C-30°C. Store away from heat and direct light.

Label

'FOR EXTERNAL USE ONLY', 'SHAKE WELL BEFORE USE', 'DO NOT TAKE BY MOUTH' and 'DO NOT FREEZE'.

Specimen Label

The specimen label for Amino Benzoic Acid Lotion BP is given as:

<table>
<tr><td colspan="3" align="center">AMINO BENZOIC ACID LOTION BP
(50 ml)</td></tr>
<tr>
<td valign="top">Composition:
Each 50 ml contains,
Amino benzoic acid - 2.5 g
Glycerin- 25 ml
Purified water q.s.- 50 ml
Dose: As directed by physician.
Storage: Store in well closed, narrow mouthed, fluted plastic bottle in cool place away from heat.</td>
<td valign="top" align="center">A-BEN LOTION
(Lotion)
Sun Protective Lotion
(Used for UV rays protection)

FOR EXTERNAL USE ONLY
SHAKE WELL BEFORE USE
DO NOT FREEZE</td>
<td valign="top">Mfg. Lic. No.- 2V/2010
Batch No.- YM 0512
Mfg. Date- Mar. 2011
Exp. Date- Feb. 2012
M.R.P.- Rs. 22.00
(Inclusive of all taxes)

Mfd. By: YAVI PHARMA
KANPUR ROAD,
LUCKNOW UP- 226001</td>
</tr>
</table>

CHAPTER 8

LINIMENTS

Liniment (or embrocation), (Latin *linere*, to anoint), is a medicated liquid topical preparation for application to the skin. This type of preparations is also called balm. Liniments are of a similar viscosity to lotions (being significantly less viscous than an ointment or cream) but unlike a lotion a liniment is applied *with friction*; that is, a liniment is always rubbed in.

Opodeldoc is a sort of liniment invented by the physician Paracelsus. *Absorbine Jr* is a trade name for a brand of liniment for human use. Traditional Chinese medicine features a wide variety of different liniments, with applications ranging from topical anaesthetics used in bone setting to simple sore muscles and bruises, such as Dit Da Jow or Ligusticum.

Liniments are alcohol or oil-based solutions that are applied externally to unbroken skin with gentle rubbing. There are two types of formulation bases that are used in the formulation of liniments: (1) alcohol-based liniments; and (2) oil-based liniments.

Alcohol-based liniments act as counterirritants and rubefacients (causing reddening of the skin) and may act to increase the penetration of the drug through the skin. In addition, these formulations will provide a cooling effect due to evaporation of the alcohol base. Examples of alcohol-based liniment are Aconite Liniment and Soap Liniment.

Conversely, oil-based liniments are employed for conditions in which a massage effect is required. Typical oils used for this purpose are arachis oil and cottonseed oil. Liniments are normally employed for the treatment of inflammatory conditions, e.g., sciatica, fibrositis and neuralgia. Examples of oil-based liniment are Methyl Salicylate Liniment BP and Camphor Liniment. In general, no other excipients are used in the formulation of liniments.

Liniments are generally used for their rubefacient, counter-irritant, mild astringent, analgesic, stimulating and penetrating effects of drugs on the external parts of the body.

Methods of Preparation

Depending on the individual ingredients, liniments are prepared in the same manner as solutions, emulsions or suspensions.

Therapeutic Uses

Liniments are typically used to relieve pain and stiffness, such as from sore muscles or from arthritis. These liniments typically are formulated from alcohol, acetone or similar quickly evaporating solvents and contain counterirritant aromatic chemical compounds such as methyl salicylate, benzoin resin or capsaicin.

Dose

The doses of different type of liniments are varied by their active ingredients e.g., the recommended dose of Methyl salicylate Liniment is 0.5 to 1 ml.

Storage Conditions

Liniments should be stored in well closed containers protected from light. Certain plastic containers, such as those made from polystyrene, are unsuitable for liniments.

Specific Labeling Requirement

The label of the liniment should state (1) the names and concentrations of the active ingredients, (2) that the liniment is intended 'FOR EXTERNAL USE ONLY', (3) if appropriate, 'SHAKE WELL BEFORE USE', (4) the date after which the liniment is not intended to be used, (5) the conditions under which the liniment should be stored, (6) the directions for using the liniment and (7) any special precautions associated with the use of the liniment.

Contraindication

Liniments should not be applied to skin areas that are broken or bruised because excessive irritation may result.

Examples of Some Liniments

1. Methyl Salicylate Liniment BP

Methyl salicylate, $C_6H_4(OH)COOCH_3$, is the methyl ester of salicylic acid, and it is the principal constituent of oil of wintergreen (about 99%). Methyl salicylate occurs as a colorless, or pale yellow, oily liquid with the strong, characteristic odor and aromatic, sweetish taste of wintergreen. It has specific gravity 1.183 to 1.188 and is optically inactive. The aqueous solution is neutral or slightly acid to litmus, and yields with a trace of ferric chloride an intense violet coloration. It is slightly soluble in water, soluble in all proportions of alcohol, ether, chloroform, glacial acetic acid, or carbon disulphide. Methyl Salicylate Liniment BP is a cutaneous emulsion. The content of methyl salicylate is 23 to 26.5% v/v in this liniment. The liniment has a characteristic odor.

Methyl salicylate is rapidly absorbed when rubbed on the skin, and this property allows the concentration of its action upon rheumatic and stiff joints and in lumbago; it may also be applied to the forearm or any convenient surface for the general action of the salicylates in acute and chronic rheumatism, pharyngitis etc. In acute lumbago, massage with methyl salicylate acts almost immediately; and it has been shown that, in the most inveterate cases of stiff back, with the presence of rheumatic nodules, such massage, applied at intervals for a month or two if necessary, will generally remove the condition. Methyl salicylate should be used for application to the skin rather than natural oil of wintergreen, as the latter frequently causes irritation and may give rise to a rubeoliform eruption.

It is recommended for local application in orchitis (inflammation of one or both testicles) and mumps. It is used as a flavoring agent, and as an antiseptic in mouth washes, tooth pastes, and powders.

Composition	Method of Preparation
Methyl salicylate- 25 ml Arachis oil q.s.- 100 ml	Take the accurately weighed methyl salicylate and dissolve in arachis oil in a closed container by agitation and immerse the container in a warm water bath. Agitate constantly to increase the solubility of methyl salicylate in arachis oil.

Label

<table>
<tr>
<td colspan="3" align="center">METHYL SALICYLATE LINIMENT BP
(50 ml)</td>
</tr>
<tr>
<td>Composition:
Each 50 ml contains,
Methyl salicylate- 12.5 ml
Arachis oil q.s.- 50 ml

Dose: As directed by the physician
Storage: Store in a tightly closed container in a cool place.</td>
<td align="center">SALICYLIN
(Liniment)
(Used in orchitis, mumps, chronic rheumatism, pharyngitis and acute lumbago)

FOR EXTERNAL USE ONLY
PROTECT FROM SUN LIGHT</td>
<td>Mfg. Lic. No.- 3J/2010
Batch No.- CK 413
Mfg. Date- June 2011
Exp. Date- May 2013
M.R.P.- Rs. 20.00
(Inclusive of all taxes)
Mfd. By: YAVI PHARMA KANPUR ROAD, LUCKNOW UP- 226001</td>
</tr>
</table>

2. Methyl Salicylate Liniment BPC

This liniment is miscible with either spirit or oil, and is used to paint over rheumatic joints or neuralgic areas, the parts being covered subsequently with flannel or gutta percha tissue.

Composition	Method of Preparation
Menthol- 5 g Oil of eucalyptus- 10 ml Essential oil of camphor- 25 ml Methyl salicylate q.s.- 100 ml	Take the accurately weighed menthol and methyl salicylate, dissolve in oil of eucalyptus and essential oil of camphor in a closed container by agitation and immerse the container in a warm water bath. Agitate constantly to increase the solubility of methyl salicylate.

Label

METHYL SALICYLATE LINIMENT BPC (50 ml)		
Composition: Each 50 ml contains, Menthol- 2.5 g Oil of eucalyptus- 5 ml Essential oil of camphor- 12.5 ml Methyl salicylate q.s.- 50 ml **Dose:** As directed by the physician **Storage:** Store in a tightly closed container in a cool place.	**METHYLIN** (Liniment) (Used in the treatment of lumbago and sciatica) **PROTECT FROM SUN LIGHT FOR EXTERNAL USE ONLY**	**Mfg. Lic. No.-** 2G/2010 **Batch No.-** NM 297 **Mfg. Date-** Apr. 2011 **Exp. Date-** Mar. 2013 **M.R.P.-** Rs. 22.00 (Inclusive of all taxes) **Mfd. By:** YAVI PHARMA KANPUR ROAD, LUCKNOW UP- 226001

3. Compound Liniment of Methyl Salicylate BPC

Composition	Method of Preparation
Menthol- 5 parts Chloral hydrate- 5 parts Extract of Indian hemp- 0.5 parts Essential oil of camphor- 25 parts Methyl salicylate q.s.- 100 parts	Dissolve the accurately weighed menthol, chloral hydrate, extract of Indian hemp, essential oil of camphor and methyl salicylate in a closed container by agitation and immerse the container in a warm water bath. Agitate constantly to increase the solubility of methyl salicylate.

Label

COMPOUND LINIMENT OF METHYL SALICYLATE BPC		
(50 ml)		
Composition: Each 50 ml contains, Menthol- 2.5 parts Chloral hydrate- 2.5 parts Extract of Indian hemp- 0.25 parts Essential oil of camphor- 12.5 parts Methyl salicylate q.s.- 50 ml **Dose:** As directed by physician. **Storage:** Store in a tightly closed container.	**MESALICYL** (Liniment) (Used in the treatment of lumbago and sciatica) **PROTECT FROM SUN LIGHT** **FOR EXTERNAL USE ONLY**	**Mfg. Lic. No.-** 5B/2010 **Batch No.-** JB 297 **Mfg. Date-** Feb. 2011 **Exp. Date-** Jan. 2012 **M.R.P.-** Rs. 25.00 (Inclusive of all taxes) **Mfd. By:** YAVI PHARMA KANPUR ROAD, LUCKNOW UP- 226001

4. White Liniment BP, BPC

White Liniment BP	White Liniment BPC (Egg Liniment)
It is a cutaneous emulsion and an extemporaneous preparation. The content of volatile oil is 24.5 to 27.5% v/w. **Composition:** Oleic acid- 85 ml Turpentine oil- 250 ml Dilute ammonia solution- 45 ml Ammonium chloride- 12.5 g Purified water q.s.- 1000 ml **Method of preparation:** Mix the required quantity of oleic acid with the turpentine oil. Dilute the dilute ammonia solution with 45 ml of the purified water, previously warmed, add to the oily solution and shake to form an emulsion. Separately dissolve the ammonium chloride in the remainder of the purified water, add to the emulsion and mix.	**Composition:** Oil of turpentine- 40 ml Acetic acid- 8.5 ml Oil of lemon- q.s. Yolk and white of egg- q.s. Distilled water q.s.- 100 ml **Method of preparation:** Mix the required quantity of oil of lemon and yolk and white of egg with the oil of turpentine. Dilute the acetic acid with 50 ml of the distilled water, previously warmed, add to the oily solution and shake to form an emulsion, make up the volume to 100 ml.

<table>
<tr><td colspan="3" align="center">Label</td></tr>
<tr><td colspan="3" align="center">WHITE LINIMENT BP
(50 ml)</td></tr>
<tr>
<td>Composition:
Each 50 ml contains,
Oleic acid- 4.25 ml
Turpentine oil- 12.5 ml
Dilute ammonia solution- 2.25 ml
Ammonium chloride- 0.625 g
Purified water q.s.- 50 ml
Storage: Store in tight container in a cool place.</td>
<td align="center">WHITELIN
(Liniment)
(Used as rubefacient and counter-irritant)

PROTECT FROM SUN LIGHT
FOR EXTERNAL USE ONLY</td>
<td>Mfg. Lic. No.- 2D/2010
Batch No.- CK 0125
Mfg. Date- May, 2011
Exp. Date- Apr. 2012
M.R.P.- Rs. 20.00
(Inclusive of all taxes)
Mfd. By: YAVI PHARMA KANPUR ROAD, LUCKNOW UP- 226001</td>
</tr>
</table>

5. Liniment of Turpentine BP

Oil of turpentine, an oleoresin is obtained by steam distillation from turpentine, obtained from *Pinus sylvestris* (Family- Coniferae), and other species of *Pinus*. It occurs as a colorless, liquid, having a strong peculiar odor, and a pungent, somewhat bitter taste, both becoming stronger and less pleasant by age and exposure to air. The odor of the French variety of turpentine oil is finer and milder than that of the American, which is terebinthinate. The sharp odor is due to an aldehyde formed by exposure of the oil to the air.

Unlike most oils, the solubility of the turpentine oil increases with age, owing to formation of more easily soluble oxidation products. The specific gravity is 0.860 to 0.870 at 25°C. The American variety is dextrorotatory and the French variety is laevorotatory. On exposure to the air it undergoes rapid change, especially in the presence of moisture. It then becomes viscid and yellow.

Oil of turpentine is rectified for medicinal purposes, and is also purified by means of lime water or solution of potassium hydroxide, any free acid being thus neutralized and removed; further, the resinified portion of the oil may be removed by shaking with alcohol and water alternately.

The oil of turpentine is antiseptic, used internally or externally, and in sufficient concentration is rapidly germicidal to all forms of bacteria. Applied to the skin it produces irritation and rubefaction, the redness being due to dilatation of the superficial vessels. Oil of turpentine is employed externally as a counter-irritant and rubefacient, in the form of Turpentine Liniment USP, Liniment of Turpentine and Acetic Acid BP and Acetic Turpentine Liniment NF in chronic rheumatism and various chest affections. To relieve deep-seated pain and inflammation, as in peritonitis (inflammation of peritoneum), flannels are wrung out of hot water, sprinkled with oil of turpentine and applied to the seat of pain.

Liniment of Turpentine BP	Turpentine Liniment USP
Composition: Soft soap- 7.5 g Camphor- 5 g Oil of turpentine- 65 ml Distilled water q.s.- 100 ml **Method of preparation:** Add 10 ml of distilled water to the soft soap, mix, and add gradually, with constant trituration, a solution of the camphor in the oil of turpentine; when the mixture thickens to a creamy consistence add sufficient distilled water to make up to the required volume.	Its specific gravity is 0.860 to 0.865 at 25°C. **Composition:** Oil of turpentine- 50 ml Sodium hydroxide q.s.- 100 ml **Method of preparation:** It is prepared by shaking oil of turpentine with an equal volume of solution of sodium hydroxide, then recovering about three-fourth of the oil by distillation, separating the clear oil from the water, and filtering.

Label

LINIMENT OF TURPENTINE BP (50 ml)		
Composition: Each 50 ml contains, Soft soap- 3.75 g Camphor- 2.5 g Oil of turpentine 32.5 ml Distilled water q.s.- 50 ml **Dose:** As directed by physician **Storage:** Store in tight container in a cool place.	**LINTURPEN** (Liniment) (Used as a rubefacient and counter-irritant) **PROTECT FROM SUN LIGHT** **FOR EXTERNAL USE ONLY**	**Mfg. Lic. No.-** 1V/2010 **Batch No.-** VM 0225 **Mfg. Date-** May, 2011 **Exp. Date-** Apr. 2012 **M.R.P.** Rs. 25.00 (Inclusive of all taxes) **Mfd. By:** YAVI PHARMA KANPUR ROAD, LUCKNOW UP- 226001

Marketed preparations

Active Ingredient(s)	Marketed Preparation (Manufacturer)
Eugenia caryophyllus	**ARHTORIL** (AVENUE L.SCIENCES)
Turpentine	**TURPENTINE LINIMENT** (GARIMA HEALTHCARE), **TURPENTINE LINIMENT** (ALPINE INDUSTRIES), **TURPENTINE LINIMENT** (ARORA PHARMACEUTICALS)
Oil of eucalyptus, camphor, menthol	**ARTHRILL** (IND-SWIFT LTD)
Methyl salicylate	**METHYL SALICYLATE** (ALPINE INDUSTRIES)

EXERCISE - 15

Object

To prepare and submit 50 ml Methyl Salicylate Liniment BP.

Theory

Liniments are alcohol- or oil-based solutions that are applied externally to unbroken skin with gentle rubbing. There are two types of formulation bases that are used in the formulation of liniments: (1) alcohol-based liniments; and (2) oil-based liniments.

Alcohol-based liniments act as counterirritants and rubefacients and may increase the penetration of the drug through the skin. In addition, these formulations will provide a cooling effect due to evaporation of the alcohol base. The oil-based liniments are employed for conditions in which a massage effect is required. Typical oils used for this purpose are arachis oil and cottonseed oil. Liniments are normally employed for the treatment of inflammatory conditions, e.g., sciatica, fibrositis and neuralgia. Methyl Salicylate Liniment BP is an example of oil-based liniment.

Methyl salicylate is the methyl ester of salicylic acid. Methyl Salicylate Liniment BP is a cutaneous emulsion. The content of methyl salicylate is 23 to 26.5% v/v in this liniment. The liniment has a characteristic odor.

Formula

Ingredients	Quantity Required
Methyl Salicylate	25 ml
Arachis oil q.s. to	100 ml

Apparatus

Glass beaker, measuring cylinder and volumetric pipette.

Procedure

Measure the required quantity of methyl salicylate and arachis oil. In this preparation arachis oil is used as a vehicle to dissolve methyl salicylate and to get a viscous preparation which is suitable to spread on the skin. Solubility of the methyl salicylate in arachis oil is further increased by heating (warming) on a water bath.

Take the accurately weighed methyl salicylate and dissolve in arachis oil in a closed container by agitation and immerse the container in a warm water bath. Agitate constantly to increase the solubility of methyl salicylate in arachis oil.

Category

Counter-irritant.

Dose

0.5 to 1 ml.

Therapeutic Use

It acts as counter-irritant for inflammed joints, sprains, rheumatic and other inflammatory conditions, also in the treatment of lumbago and sciatica.

Storage

Methyl Salicylate Liniment BP should be stored in a narrow mouthed, light-resistant glass bottle and should be tightly closed with a plastic screw cap and supplied with an applicator. High temperature may cause the volatilization of methyl salicylate hence it should be stored in a cool place.

Label

The label should have the caution 'FOR EXTERNAL USE ONLY', 'NOT TO BE APPLIED ON WOUNDS AND BROKEN SKIN', 'SHAKE WELL BEFORE USE' and 'STORE IN A COOL PLACE'.

Specimen Label

The specimen label for Methyl Salicylate Liniment BP is given as:

<table>
<tr><td colspan="3" align="center">METHYL SALICYLATE LINIMENT BP
(50 ml)</td></tr>
<tr>
<td valign="top">Composition:
Each 50 ml contains,
Methyl salicylate- 12.5 ml
Arachis oil q.s.- 50 ml
Dose: 0.5 to 1 ml
Storage: Store in a narrow mouthed, tightly closed, light-resistant glass bottle in cool place.
(Not to be applied on wounds and broken skin)</td>
<td valign="top" align="center">MESALICYL
(Liniment)
Counter-irritant
(used in inflammed joints, sprains, rheumatic and other inflammatory conditions)

FOR EXTERNAL USE ONLY
SHAKE WELL BEFORE USE</td>
<td valign="top">Mfg. Lic. No.- 4H/2010
Batch No.- UJ 0510
Mfg. Date- July 2011
Exp. Date- June 2012
M.R.P.- Rs. 25.00
(Inclusive of all taxes)

Mfd. By: YAVI PHARMA KANPUR ROAD, LUCKNOW UP- 226001</td>
</tr>
</table>

EXERCISE - 16

Object

To prepare and submit 50 ml Turpentine Liniment BP.

Theory

Liniments are alcohol- or oil-based solutions that are applied externally to unbroken skin with gentle rubbing. There are two types of liniments: alcohol-based liniments and oil-based liniments.

Turpentine oil is a volatile oil obtained from distillation of turpentine which is an oleo resin obtained from various species of *pinus*. Turpentine is not miscible with water and it does not contain any free fatty acids so it can not form soap with alkaline substances. Therefore soft soap (monovalent soap, alkaline in nature) is used which also act as emulsifying agent.

Camphor is soluble in turpentine oil hence biphasic system can be prepared using soft soap which produces o/w type of emulsion. In this preparation turpentine oil remains as dispersed phase and water as continuous phase.

Formula

Ingredients	Quantity Required
Soft soap	7.5 g
Camphor	5 g
Oil of turpentine (freshly rectified)	65 ml
Purified water q.s. to	100 ml

Apparatus

Glass beaker, measuring cylinder and volumetric pipette.

Procedure

Measure the required quantity of all ingredients. In a dried container dissolve camphor in freshly rectified turpentine oil. Mix the soft soap with small amount of purified water (10 ml). Gradually add camphor solution to the soap mixture with trituration until a thick creamy emulsion is formed. Allow it to stand for few minutes for the separation of air bubbles. Then add sufficient amount of purified water to make up the volume 100 ml and mix well.

Category

Rubefacient and counter-irritant.

Dose

1 to 2 ml.

Therapeutic Use

It acts as counter-irritant and rubefacient and it is mainly used in patients suffering from arthralgia (pain in joints), myalgia (muscular pain), fibrocitis (ligamental pain) and sprain.

Storage

It should be stored in well-closed, narrow mouthed light resistant glass container in cool place to prevent the volatilization of camphor.

Turpentine oil undergoes rapid changes when comes in contact with air and moisture so the container should be close tightly with a plastic screw cap and supplied with an applicator.

Label

The label should have the caution 'PROTECT FROM SUN LIGHT' with red ink due to the presence of volatile constituents in the preparation. The label should also have the directions 'FOR EXTERNAL USE ONLY', 'NOT TO BE APPLIED ON WOUNDS AND BROKEN SKIN', 'SHAKE WELL BEFORE USE' and 'STORE IN A COOL AND DRY PLACE'.

Caution

On exposure to air, turpentine oil undergoes rapid changes especially in the presence of moisture and becomes viscous yellow and acidic reactions take place. Therefore freshly rectified turpentine oil should be used for the preparation of liniment.

Specimen Label

The specimen label for Methyl salicylate liniment BP is given as:

<table>
<tr><td colspan="3" align="center">TURPENTINE LINIMENT BP
(50 ml)</td></tr>
<tr>
<td valign="top">

Composition:

Each 50 ml contains,

Soft soap- 37.5 g

Camphor- 2.5 g

Oil of turpentine- 32.5 ml

Purified water q.s.- 50 ml

Dose: 1 to 2 ml

Storage: Store in a narrow mouthed, tightly closed, light-resistant glass bottle in cool place.

</td>
<td valign="top" align="center">

TURPELIN

(Liniment)

Rubefacient and Counterirritant

(Used in joint pain, muscular pain and ligamental pain)

FOR EXTERNAL USE ONLY

SHAKE WELL BEFORE USE

</td>
<td valign="top">

Mfg. Lic. No.- 4H/2010

Batch No.- CK 0125

Mfg. Date- July 2011

Exp. Date- June 2012

M.R.P.- Rs. 25.00

(Inclusive of all taxes)

Mfd. By: YAVI PHARMA

KANPUR ROAD, LUCKNOW

UP- 226001

(Not to be applied on wounds and broken skin)

</td>
</tr>
</table>

CHAPTER 9

MUCILAGES

Mucilages are thick, viscid, adhesive liquids, produced by dispersing gum in water, or by extracting the mucilaginous ingredients from vegetable substances with water. All mucilages are prone to decomposition, showing appreciable decrease in viscosity on storage. They should never be made in quantities larger than can be used immediately, unless a preservative is added.

Both acacia and tragacanth either are partially or completely insoluble in alcohol. Tragacanth is precipitated from solution by alcohol, but acacia is soluble in diluted alcoholic solutions. Several synthetic mucilage-like substances such as polyvinyl alcohol, methylcellulose, carboxymethylcellulose, are used as mucilage substitutes at the appropriate concentration.

Acacia gum is a dried exudate from *Acacia senegal* (Family- Leguminosae). It forms viscous solutions in water. On storage the mucilage becomes acidic due to enzyme action and since its viscosity falls sharply below pH 4, deterioration occurs rapidly. Acacia also contains an oxidase enzyme that causes deterioration of easily oxidized medicaments.

Tragacanth is a dried extract from *Astragalus gummifer* (Family- Leguminosae). With water it forms viscous solution or gel depending on the concentration. As with acacia, the mucilage should be used only if the vehicle of the suspension is water or chloroform water. Tragacanth produces less sticky mucilage than acacia hence it is more suitable for external preparations.

Sodium alginate mainly consists of sodium salts of alginic acid, a polyuronic acid from seaweed, Laminaria. It forms a viscous solution with water, about 1% giving a product with approximately the same suspending power as tragacanth mucilage. Alginate mucilages are most viscous about an hour after preparation after which there is a fall to a

113

fairly constant value at about 24 hours. Hence they should be allowed to stand overnight before use. Maximum viscosity is at about pH 7 and at pH 4 and 10 it is only 10% lower. Sodium alginate is less variable in composition than the natural gums and therefore its mucilages are more uniform in viscosity.

Methylcellulose is partly o-methylated cellulose. It may be represented by $[C_6H_7O_2(OH)_2OCH_3]_n$ where n may be about 1000. Methylcellulose mucilages are clear or opalescent, colorless, tasteless, odorless, inert and neutral. They keep well for many months at room temperature but, although they are less susceptible to microbial attack than natural gums, a preservative e.g. phenylmercuric nitrate (0.001%), should be added. They are nonionic therefore stable over a wide pH range.

On heating, these mucilages first decrease in viscosity and then as the temperature rises, the methylcellulose molecules gradually become dehydrated until, at about 50°C the dispersion gels. On cooling, the gel reverts to a sol and the viscosity returns to normal.

Methylcellulose Oral Solution USP is a flavored solution. It may be prepared by adding slowly the methylcellulose to one-third the amount of boiling water, with stirring, until it is thoroughly wetted, then cold water should be added and the wetted material allowed to dissolve while stirring. The viscosity of the solution will depend upon the concentration and the specification of the methylcellulose.

Methods of Preparation

Uniformly smooth mucilages sometimes are difficult to prepare because of the uneven wetting of the gums. In general, it is best to use fine gum particles and disperse them with agitation in a small quantity of 95% alcohol or in cold water (except for methylcellulose). Then the appropriate amount of water can be added with constant stirring.

Tragacanth mucilage can be prepared from the flakes or powder but latter is easier to use. Flakes give more viscous products. The powders that have been over heated during milling or stored for a long time give mucilage of low viscosity. Tragacanth contains a soluble and insoluble fraction; the insoluble fraction hydrates rather slowly and consequently, mucilages increase significantly in viscosity for a time after preparation and it is an advantage not to use them for a few days. Beyond the pH range 4 - 7.5, they lose viscosity quickly. Mucilages must be preserved if long storage is desired.

In preparation of sodium alginate mucilage, the mucilage lumps are prevented by using 2-4% alcohol, glycerin or propylene glycol as dispersing agent. Alternatively the vehicle may be mechanically stirred while the powder is slowly sprinkled into the vertex.

Warming the vehicle hastens solution but temperatures above 70°C cause depolymerization with consequent loss of viscosity.

Therapeutic Uses

Mucilages are used primarily to aid in suspending insoluble substances in liquids; their colloidal nature and viscosity help prevent immediate sedimentation. Methylcellulose is used widely as a bulk laxative because it absorbs water and swells to a hydrogel in the intestine in similar manner as psyllium or karaya gum. Methylcellulose is used both in internal and external preparations in concentration between 0.5-2%. Tragacanth mucilage is used in jellies, lotions, pastes and creams. The synthetic gums are non-glycogenic and may be used in the preparation of diabetic syrups.

Dose

The dose of mucilages is usually 15 to 30 ml.

Storage Conditions

Mucilages are susceptible to microbial attack so for the long time storage of mucilages, a preservative must be added e.g., in methylcellulose mucilages a preservative phenylmercuric nitrate (concentration 0.001%) should be added. In case of acacia mucilage an antimicrobial agent is necessary. Chloroform, benzoic acid and parahydroxybenzoic acid (PABA) esters are suitable but if chloroform is used, the mucilage soon becomes foul if it is not stored in well-closed containers in a cool place to prevent the loss of the preservative by volatilization.

Specific Labeling Requirement

'SHAKE WELL BEFORE USE', 'DO NOT FREEZE'.

Contraindication

Methylcellulose mucilage is incompatible with chlorocresol, phenol, resorcinol, tannic acid, acridines and silver nitrate by producing turbidity and loss of viscosity.

Sodium alginate is an anionic compound and is incompatible with cationic antiseptics, like acridines, crystal violet and cetrimide. It is also incompatible with heavy metals, calcium salts and phenylmercuric salts.

Examples of Some Mucilage

1. Acacia Mucilage

In Acacia Mucilage, acacia tears should be used because powder gives an opalescent preparation.

Composition	Method of Preparation
Acacia (in tears)- 40 g Chloroform water- 60 ml Chloroform water (double strength)- 100 ml Purified water- 100 ml	Put the acacia tears in a beaker and remove surface impurities by rinsing well with chloroform water. Transfer the acacia tears in the bag of muslin cloth and suspend the bag in chloroform water. The acacia tears should be hanged in the vehicle without touching the bottom of the jar. Leave 2-3 days until the solution is complete, squeeze the bag and stir the product gently. This method has several advantages like the acacia tears do not adhere to the jar so their separation is easy; the muslin cloth collects impurities from the acacia tears thus eliminating the final straining process. This is a stock preparation, not intended for issue to a patient.

Label

ACACIA MUCILAGE (50 ml)		
Composition: Each 50 ml contains, Acacia- 20 g Chloroform water- 30 ml Chloroform water (double strength)- 50 ml Purified water- 50 ml **Storage:** Store in tightly closed container.	**ACACILAGE** (Mucilage) (Used as thickening agent and suspending agent) **SHAKE WELL BEFORE USE**	**Mfg. Lic. No.-** 5H/2010 **Batch No.-** AC 297 **Mfg. Date-** June 2011 **Exp. Date-** Dec. 2011 **M.R.P.-** Rs. 18.00 (Inclusive of all taxes) **Mfd. By:** YAVI PHARMA KANPUR ROAD, LUCKNOW UP- 226001

2. Tragacanth Mucilage BPC

Like Acacia Mucilage, it is also a stock preparation. Tragacanth powder is used because solution of the flakes is very poor. Addition of tragacanth to water or vice versa gives a lumpy product due to the agglomeration of the sticky, poorly wettable particles. To obtain a homogeneous preparation a liquid that is poorly absorbed by the gum is needed. For this purpose alcohol is used but glycerin and essential oils are suitable alternatives for preparations.

Composition	Method of Preparation	Caution
Tragacanth (finely powdered)- 12.5 g Alcohol (90%)- 12 ml Chloroform water q.s.- 1000 ml	Put the required amount of alcohol in wide-mouthed jar and then add tragacanth. Agitate to mix. Hold the jar over the sink and pour in the 95 ml of vehicle as quickly as possible.	The addition of alcohol to the tragacanth may lead to lumpiness.

Label

<table>
<tr><td colspan="3" align="center">TRAGACANTH MUCILAGE BPC
(50 ml)</td></tr>
<tr>
<td>Composition:
Each 50 ml contains,
Tragacanth (finely powdered)- 0.625 g
Alcohol (90%)- 0.6 ml
Chloroform water q.s.- 50 ml
Storage: Store in tightly closed container in a cool place.</td>
<td align="center">TRAGACILAGE
(Mucilage)
(Used as thickening and suspending agent)

SHAKE WELL BEFORE USE
DO NOT FREEZE</td>
<td>Mfg. Lic. No.- 2D/2010
Batch No.- GH 297
Mfg. Date- Apr. 2011
Exp. Date- Oct. 2012
M.R.P.- Rs. 20.00
(Inclusive of all taxes)
Mfd. By: YAVI PHARMA KANPUR ROAD, LUCKNOW UP- 226001</td>
</tr>
</table>

3. Starch Mucilage BPC

Starch Mucilage BPC is a stock preparation. It must be freshly prepared because it does not contain any preservative.

Composition	Method of Preparation
Starch- 25 g Purified water q.s.- 1000 ml	Boil purified water (160 ml) in a 500 ml wide-mouthed conical flask. In a mortar triturate the required quantity of starch with about 30 ml of purified water. Pour this suspension into the boiling water and shake. Keep the preparation hot while the mortar is rinsed with rest of the purified water. Reheat to boiling with frequent agitation. The starch becomes gelatinized and forms mucilage, which should be free from lumps. Remove from the heat and immediately cool the flask by rotating under the stream of cool water. This prevents formation of a skin. Measure and make up the volume with purified water which is lost by evaporation.

Label

STARCH MUCILAGE BPC **(50 ml)**		
Composition: Each 50 ml contains, Starch- 1.25 g Purified water q.s.- 50 ml **Storage:** Store in a tightly closed container in a cool place.	**STARCILAGE** (Mucilage) (Used as emollient and lubricating agent for catheters) **SHAKE WELL BEFORE USE** **DO NOT FREEZE**	**Mfg. Lic. No.-** 5M/2010 **Batch No.-** CK 297 **Mfg. Date-** Aug. 2011 **Exp. Date-** Feb. 2012 **M.R.P.-** Rs. 15.00 (Inclusive of all taxes) **Mfd. By:** YAVI PHARMA KANPUR ROAD, LUCKNOW UP- 226001

Marketed preparations

No preparation is available in the market.

EXERCISE - 17

Object

To prepare and submit 50 ml Starch Mucilage IP.

Theory

The official mucilages are thick, viscid, adhesive liquid produced by dispersing gum in water or by extracting the mucilaginous material from vegetable substances with water. All the mucilages are prone to decomposition showing appreciable decrease in viscosity on storage. They should never be made in quantities larger than can be used immediately, unless a preservative is added.

Starch consists of polysaccharide granules obtained from the caryopsis (structure of one seeded fruit in which ovary wall is attached with seed coat) of maize or corn (*Zea mays*), or of rice (*Oryza sativa*), or of wheat (*Triticum aestivum*), or from the tuber of potato (*Solanum tuberosum*) or from the rhizomes of tapioca (*Manihot utilissima*).

Uniformly smooth mucilages sometimes are difficult to prepare because of the uneven wetting of the gums. In general, it is best to use fine gum particles and disperse them with good agitation in a little 95% alcohol or in cold water (except for methyl cellulose) the appropriate amount of water that can be added with the constant stirring.

Microbial limit

1 g of starch mucilage should be free from *Escherichia coli* and *Salmonellae.*

Formula

Ingredients	Quantity Required
Starch	2 g
Purified water q.s. to	100 ml

Apparatus

Glass beaker and measuring cylinder.

Procedure

Weigh the required quantity of starch. Prepare the suspension of starch in 100 ml of purified water, boil for 1 minute and cool; thin and cloudy mucilage is produced with all starches except potato starch which gives thick and more transparent mucilage. Transfer in clean amber colored glass container and close it tightly.

Category

Pharmaceutical aid.

Dose

10 to 20 ml

Therapeutic Use

Mucilages are used primarily to aid in suspending the insoluble substances in liquids, their colloidal character and viscosity help to prevent immediate sedimentation.

Storage

Starch Mucilage IP should be stored in well-closed, light resistant container in cool place.

Label

The label should have the caution 'STORE IN A DARK AND COOL PLACE'.

Specimen Label

The specimen label for Starch mucilage IP is given as:

<table>
<tr><td colspan="3" align="center">STARCH MUCILAGE IP
(50 ml)</td></tr>
<tr>
<td>Composition:
Each 50 ml contains,
Starch- 1 g
Purified water q.s.-50 ml
Dose: 15 to 30 ml
Storage: Store in well-closed container in cool place.</td>
<td align="center">STARLAGE
(Mucilage)
(Used as Suspending Agent)

SHAKE WELL BEFORE USE
STORE IN A DARK PLACE</td>
<td>Mfg. Lic. No.- 2M/2010
Batch No.- CQ 0512
Mfg. Date- May 2011
Exp. Date- Nov. 2012
M.R.P.- Rs. 14.00
(Inclusive of all taxes)
Mfd. By: YAVI PHARMA
KANPUR ROAD,
LUCKNOW UP- 226001</td>
</tr>
</table>

CHAPTER 10

GLYCERINS/GLYCERITES

Glycerins or glycerites are solutions or mixtures of medicinal substances in not less than 50% by weight of glycerin. Glycerine is a colorless, odorless, viscous liquid that is widely used in pharmaceutical formulations. Glycerol has three hydrophilic hydroxyl groups that are responsible for its solubility in water and its hygroscopic nature. It is sweet-tasting and of low toxicity. Most of the glycerins are extremely viscous and some are of jelly like consistency. Glycerin is a valuable pharmaceutical solvent forming permanent and concentrated solutions not otherwise obtainable.

Glycerin is a trihydric alcohol and is miscible with both water and alcohol. It is rated as one of the most valuable products known to pharmacy due to its solvent and preservative properties. It is also useful as an emollient and humectant. Glycerin is an essential ingredient of products like throat paints due to its viscosity.

Glycerin is a good solvent for many substances which are not very soluble in water e.g., borax and phenol. It also acts as a preservative. It also extracts large quantities of tannins and their oxidation products when these are present in drug. Its low volatility and hygroscopic character are of value in maintaining preparations such as kaolin poultice in a moist condition. As noted under otic solutions, glycerin alone is used to aid in the removal of cerumen.

Glycerin can be used undiluted, in a small quantity, as a rectal injection or suppository to immediately relieve constipation. When mixed half and half with rosewater, it provides a good skin emollient. Glycerin is soothing to the skin, and moisturizes without feeling greasy. When mixed with 25% alcohol, it can be applied to acne, acting as a strong drawing agent. When mixed with 25% water, it helps relieve itching skin.

A glycerite is a fluid extract of an herb or other medicinal substance made using glycerin as being integral to the fluid extraction medium. Glycerites that contain adequate glycerin concentration, especially approaching 70%, do not allow for microbial growth, and, in fact, are excellent microbial suppressants.

Methods of Preparation

Since glycerol forms the backbone of triglycerides, it is produced by saponification of animal fats e.g., a byproduct of soap-making. It is also a byproduct of the production of biodiesel via trans-esterification.

For the preparation of glycerite, pour herbs (finely chopped, ground, or powdered) into a clean jar. Measure the glycerin and add distilled water to it. Pour the glycerin/water mixture over the herbs. Macerate for at least two weeks, agitating daily. Essential oils can be added to a glycerite to enhance the flavor and aroma. Tangerine, orange, lemon and mint oils are especially popular. Glycerites are frequently used as a substitute for alcohol in tinctures.

Therapeutic Uses

Glycerol is used in medical, pharmaceutical and personal care preparations, mainly as a means of improving smoothness, providing lubrication and as a humectant. It is found in cough syrups, elixirs, expectorants, toothpaste, mouthwashes, skin care products, shaving cream, hair care products, soaps and water based personal lubricants. Used as a laxative when introduced into the rectum in suppository or small-volume (2 to10 ml) as enema form; irritates the anal mucosa and induces a hyperosmotic effect. Glycerol is a component of glycerol soap. Topical pure or nearly pure glycerol is an effective treatment for psoriasis, burns, bites, cuts, rashes, bedsores and calluses. It can be used orally to eliminate halitosis (unpleasing smelling breath), as it is a contact bacterial desiccant. The same property makes it very helpful with periodontal disease; it penetrates biofilm quickly and eliminates bacterial colonies.

Dose

As directed by physician.

Storage Conditions

Glycerins are hygroscopic in nature so it should be stored in tightly closed containers in cool place.

Specific Labeling Requirement

'SHAKE WELL BEFORE USE'.

Examples of Some Glycerite

1. Glycerite

Composition	Method of Preparation
Herbs (finely chopped or powdered)- 50 g Distilled water-320 ml Glycerin q.s.- 1000 ml	Pour herbs into a clean jar. Measure out glycerin and add distilled water to it. Pour the glycerin/water mixture over the herbs. Macerate for at least two weeks, agitating daily.

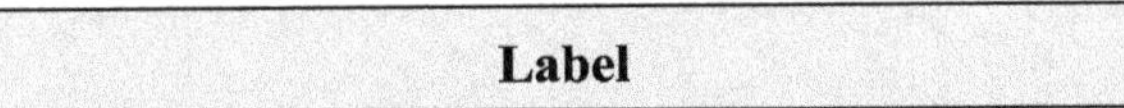

GLYCERITE (50 ml)		
Composition: Each 50 ml contains, Herbs (powdered)- 2.5 g Distilled water- 16 ml Glycerin q.s.- 50 ml **Storage:** Store in a tightly closed container.	**HERBGLY** (Glycerite) (Used as protectant) **PROTECT FROM SUN LIGHT FOR EXTERNAL USE ONLY**	**Mfg. Lic. No.-** 3M/2010 **Batch No.-** AS 524 **Mfg. Date-** July 2011 **Exp. Date-** May 2012 **M.R.P.-** Rs. 21.00 (Inclusive of all taxes) **Mfd. By:** YAVI PHARMA KANPUR ROAD, LUCKNOW UP- 226001

2. Echinacea and Orange Glycerite

It is used at the first sign of a cold or flu. This glycerite helps stave off colds or the flu. If illness sets in, increase the dose to 1-3 droppersful every few hours for about a week. For children, half the dosage, depending on the child's height and weight.

Composition	Method of Preparation
Echinacea (dried flowers and leaves)- 45 g Honey- 30 ml Essential oil (orange, tangerine, or cinnamon)- 20-30 drops Vegetable glycerin- 237 ml	Put herb and glycerin into a blender and whirl until smooth. Pour into a clean jar and keep in a warm place. Shake daily for 2 to 3 weeks. Pour contents into a muslin bag and squeeze out the liquid, discarding the herbs. If desired, add honey and essential oil. Mix well and put into small amber bottles with droppers.

Label

ECHINACEA AND ORANGE GLYCERITE (50 ml)		
Composition: Each 50 ml contains, Echinacea- 9 g Honey- 6 ml Essential oil- q.s. Vegetable glycerin q.s.- 50 ml **Dose:** One to three droppersful 3 or 4 times a day for 7 to 10 days, away from meals. **Storage:** Store in a tightly closed container.	**ECHIORA** (Glycerite) (Used in cold or flu) **PROTECT FROM SUN LIGHT** **SHAKE WELL BEFORE USE**	**Mfg. Lic. No.-** 5F/2010 **Batch No.-** CL 153 **Mfg. Date-** Apr. 2011 **Exp. Date-** Mar. 2012 **M.R.P.-** Rs. 22.00 (Inclusive of all taxes) **Mfd. By:** YAVI PHARMA KANPUR ROAD, LUCKNOW UP- 226001

3. Glycerin and Gelatin Base BP

Composition	Method of Preparation
Gelatin (powdered)- 14 g Glycerin- 70 ml Purified water q.s.- 100 ml	With a whisk, blend the glycerin and water together in the top of a double boiler (adding water to the bottom). Stir in the gelatin and heat the mixture over a medium-high heat until it turns clear. Pour into a shallow glass pan to set.

Label

GLYCERIN AND GELATIN BASE BP (50 ml)		
Composition: Each 50 ml contains, Gelatin (powdered)- 7 g Vegetable glycerin- 35 ml Purified water q.s.- 50 ml **Storage:** Store in a tightly closed container.	**GELACERIN** (Glycerite) (Used as a base for suppositories, pessaries, and pastilles) **PROTECT FROM SUN LIGHT**	**Mfg. Lic. No.-** 1W/2010 **Batch No.-** AL 243 **Mfg. Date-** Apr. 2011 **Exp. Date-** Oct. 2012 **M.R.P.-** Rs. 17.00 (Inclusive of all taxes) **Mfd. By:** YAVI PHARMA KANPUR ROAD, LUCKNOW UP- 226001

4. Borax Glycerin IP

Composition	Method of Preparation
Borax- 12 g Glycerin q.s- 100 g	Powder the borax. Triturate the required quantity of fine powder of borax with glycerin. Warm the mixture with constant stirring until borax is dissolved, filter it, if necessary.

Label

<table>
<tr><td colspan="3" align="center">BORAX GLYCERIN IP
(50 g)</td></tr>
<tr>
<td>Composition:
Each 50 g contains,
Borax- 6 g
Glycerin q.s.- 50 g
Storage: Store in a tightly closed container.</td>
<td align="center">BORGYL
(Glycerite)
(Used as bacteriostatic)

PROTECT FROM SUN LIGHT
SHAKE WELL BEFORE USE</td>
<td>Mfg. Lic. No.- 5A/2010
Batch No.- BH 013
Mfg. Date- Nov. 2011
Exp. Date- Oct. 2012
M.R.P.- Rs. 27.00
(Inclusive of all taxes)
Mfd. By: YAVI PHARMA KANPUR ROAD, LUCKNOW UP- 226001</td>
</tr>
</table>

5. Tannic acid Glycerin IP

Composition	Method of Preparation
Tannic acid- 20 g Sodium citrate- 1 g Sodium sulphate- 0.2 g Glycerin q.s.-100 g	Powder the ingredients. Triturate the required quantity of tannic acid, sodium citrate and sodium sulphate with half quantity of glycerin until a smooth paste is formed. Add the remaining quantity of glycerin. Warm the mixture with occasional stirring until a homogeneous solution is obtained.

Label

<table>
<tr><td colspan="3" align="center">TANNIC ACID GLYCERIN IP
(50 g)</td></tr>
<tr>
<td>

Composition:

Each 50 g contains,

Tannic acid- 10 g

Sodium citrate- 0.5 g

Sodium sulphate- 0.1 g

Glycerin q.s.-50 g

Storage: Store in a tightly closed container.

</td>
<td align="center">

TANGYL

(Glycerite)

(Used as astringent and antiseptic)

FOR EXTERNAL USE ONLY

SHAKE WELL BEFORE USE

</td>
<td>

Mfg. Lic. No.- 2L/2010

Batch No.- SG 045

Mfg. Date- Sep. 2011

Exp. Date- Aug. 2012

M.R.P.- Rs. 25.00

(Inclusive of all taxes)

Mfd. By: YAVI PHARMA KANPUR ROAD, LUCKNOW UP- 226001

</td>
</tr>
</table>

Marketed Preparations

Active Ingredient(s)	Marketed Preparation (Manufacturer)
Tannic acid and glycerin	**GUMEX** (PHARMADENT), **SENSOFORM** (INDOCO), **STOLIN GUM ASTRINGENT** (DR. REDDY'S LAB), **S.G.PAINT** (CENTAUR)
Borax, tannic acid and glycerin	**GUM CORRECT** (EPIC PHARMACEUTICALS)

EXERCISE - 18

Object

To prepare and submit 50 g Kaolin Poultice BP.

Theory

Poultices are also known as cataplasms. These are ancient class of semisolid preparations meant for external application. Poultices are soft, viscous, paste like wet masses of medicament and other solid ingredients applied to the skin while they are hot, to reduce the inflammation, pain or to act as counter irritant.

Poultices are applied when they are hot because they stimulate body surface or improve an inflamed area by supplying the medicament in the presence of heat. Heavy kaolin is commonly used in the preparation of poultice because it acts as a carrier of heat. Kaolin is a good absorbent, which absorbs infectious and watery material. Glycerin is hygroscopic in nature hence it withdraws exudates from infected tissues. Boric acid acts as an antiseptic. Methyl salicylate and thymol act as counter irritant while peppermint oil is used as perfume.

Kaolin is liable to be contaminated with spores of *Clostridium tetani* hence it is necessary to heat up to 120°C for 1 hour to kill these spores.

Formula

Ingredients	Quantity Required
Heavy kaolin (finely sifted)	527 g
Boric acid (finely sifted)	45 g
Methyl salicylate	2 ml
Thymol	0.5 g
Peppermint oil	0.5 ml
Glycerol	425 g

Apparatus

Glass beaker, measuring cylinder and volumetric pipette.

Procedure

Measure the required quantity of all ingredients. Mix the heavy kaolin, previously dried at 100°C and the boric acid with the glycerol, heat at 120°C for 1 hour, stirring occasionally and allows to cool. Separately, dissolve the thymol in the methyl salicylate, add to the cooled mixture then add the peppermint oil and mix thoroughly.

Note : The heating step may be omitted if some other satisfactory means of mixing the solid ingredients with the glycerol is used but in that case heavy kaolin (previously sterilized) is used.

Category

Cataplasm.

Dose

5 to 10 g spread thickly on dressing material or lint and apply to the affected area as hot as the patient can bear the temperature.

Therapeutic Use

Due to the absorptive and hygroscopic nature of Kaolin Poultice BP, it is used for the treatment of boils and similar infections. For application, poultice is heated along with the container with occasional stirring until it can only just be tolerated on the back of the hand then hot mass is spread thickly on dressing material and applied to the affected area as hot as the patient can bear the temperature. Kaolin Poultice BP is used to reduce inflammation, pain and drain out the infectious material from the diseased tissues. It is also used as counter irritant.

Storage

Since thymol, methyl salicylate and peppermint oil are volatile in nature and glycerin absorbs moisture from atmosphere hence Kaolin Poultice BP should be stored in a thermo resistant soda lime glass bottle or container made up of tin and tightly closed with metallic screwed cap lined with impermeable layer. The Kaolin Poultice BP should be stored in cool place to prevent the evaporation of volatile ingredients.

Label

If poultice is supplied in tin container then on the label caution should be given to the patient as 'LOOSEN THE LID BEFORE HEATING'. If poultice is supplied in a glass container then caution is given as 'TRANSFER THE REQUIRED AMOUNT OF POULTICE TO CHINA DISH AND HEAT TO AVOID BREAKING OF GLASS CONTAINER FROM DIRECT HEATING'. Poultice should bear direction on the label, 'Heat the preparation and spread thickly on dressing material or lint and apply to the affected area as hot as the patient can bear the temperature'.

Along with general requirements of label poultice should bear auxiliary label as 'FOR EXTERNAL USE ONLY', 'STORE IN COOL PLACE'.

Specimen Label

The specimen label for Kaolin Poultice BP is given as:

<table>
<tr><td colspan="3" align="center">KAOLIN POULTICE BP
(50 g)</td></tr>
<tr>
<td>Composition:
Each 50 g contains,
Heavy kaolin- 26.35 g
Boric acid- 2.25 g
Methyl salicylate- 0.1 ml
Thymol- 0.025 g
Peppermint oil- 0.025 ml
Glycerol- 21.25 g
Dose: 5 to 10 g
Heat the preparation and spread thickly on dressing material or lint and apply to the affected area as hot as the patient can bear the temperature.</td>
<td align="center">YAKA POULTICE
(Poultice)
Cataplasm
(for the treatment of boils and similar infections)

FOR EXTERNAL USE ONLY</td>
<td>Mfg. Lic. No.- 2C/2010
Batch No.- YV 0205
Mfg. Date- Aug. 2011
Exp. Date- July 2012
M.R.P.- Rs. 28.00
(Inclusive of all taxes)
Storage- Store in well closed tin container in cool place.
Mfd. By: YAVI PHARMA
KANPUR ROAD, LUCKNOW UP- 226001</td>
</tr>
</table>

CHAPTER 11

INHALATIONS

Inhalations are liquid or solid preparations intended for administration as vapors or aerosols to the lung in order to obtain a local or systemic effect. They contain one or more active substances which may be dissolved or dispersed in a suitable vehicle. Inhalations may, depending on the type of preparation, contain propellants, co-solvents, diluents, antimicrobial preservatives, solubilizing and stabilizing agents, etc. These excipients do not adversely affect the functions of the mucosa of the respiratory tract or its cilia. Inhalations are intended to release volatile constituents for inhalation either when placed on a pad or when added to hot (not boiling) water.

According to the USP, inhalations are the drugs or solutions or suspensions of one or more drug substances administered to the nasal or oral respiratory route for local or systemic effects. Solutions of drug substances in sterile water for inhalation or in sodium chloride inhalation solution may be nebulized by the use of inert gases. Nebulizers are suitable for the administration of inhalation solutions only if they give droplets sufficiently fine and uniform in size so that the mist reaches the bronchioles. Nebulized solutions may be breathed directly from the nebulizer or the nebulizer may be attached to a plastic face mask or intermittent positive pressure breathing machine.

Inhalation solution and suspension drug products are typically aqueous-based formulations that contain therapeutically active ingredients and can also contain additional excipients. Aqueous-based oral inhalation solutions and suspension must be sterile. Inhalation solutions and suspensions are intended for delivery to the lungs by oral inhalation for local or systemic effects and are used with a specified nebulizer. Unit-dose presentation is recommended for these drug products to prevent microbial contamination during use. The container closure system for these drug products consists of the container and closure and can include protective packaging such as foil overwrap.

Preparations intended to be administered as aerosols (dispersions of solid or liquid particles in a gas) are administered by one of the following devices: nebulizer, pressurized metered-dose inhaler, dry-powder inhaler. Inhalations are supplied in multidose or single-dose containers. When supplied in pressurized containers, they comply with the requirements of the pressurized pharmaceutical preparations.

129

An inhalation spray drug product consists of the formulation and the container closure system. The formulations are typically aqueous based and do not contain any propellant. Aqueous-based oral inhalation sprays must be sterile. Inhalation sprays are intended for delivery to the lungs by oral inhalation for local or systemic effects. The products contain therapeutically active ingredients and can also contain additional excipients. The formulation can be in unit-dose or multi-dose presentations. The use of preservatives or stabilizing agents in inhalation spray formulations is discouraged. If these excipients are included in a formulation, their use should be justified by assessment in a clinical setting to ensure the safety and tolerability of the drug product. The dose is delivered by the integral pump components of the container closure system to the lungs by oral inhalation for local or systemic effects.

A special class of inhalations termed inhalants consists of drugs or combination of drugs that by virtue of their high vapor pressure can be carried by an air current into the nasal passage where they exert their effect. The container from which the inhalant generally is administered is known as an inhaler. The preparations which are used for the inhalations may be liquid or powder.

1. Liquid Preparations for Inhalation

Three categories of liquid preparations for inhalation may be distinguished:
   (A) Preparations intended to be converted into vapor,
   (B) Liquid preparations for nebulization,
   (C) Pressurized metered-dose preparations for inhalation.

Liquid preparations for inhalation are solutions or dispersions. Dispersions are readily dispersible on shaking and they remain sufficiently stable to enable the correct dose to be delivered. Suitable excipients may be used.

(A) Preparations Intended to be Converted into Vapor

These preparations are intended to be converted into vapor are solutions, dispersions or solid preparations. They are usually added to hot water and the vapor generated is inhaled.

(B) Liquid Preparations for Nebulization

Liquid preparations for inhalation intended to be converted into aerosols by continuously operating nebulizers or metered-dose nebulizers are solutions, suspensions or emulsions. Suitable co-solvents or solubilizers may be used to increase the solubility of the active substances. Liquid preparations for nebulization in concentrated form for use in continuously operating nebulizers are diluted to the prescribed volume with the prescribed liquid before use. Liquids for nebulization may also be prepared from powders. The pH of the liquid preparations for use in continuously operating nebulizers is not lower than 3 and not higher than 8.5.

Suspensions and emulsions are readily dispersible on shaking and they remain sufficiently stable to enable the correct dose to be delivered. Aqueous preparations for nebulization supplied in multi-dose containers may contain a suitable antimicrobial preservative at a suitable concentration except where the preparation itself has adequate antimicrobial properties.

Continuously operating nebulizers are devices that convert liquids into aerosols by high-pressure gases, ultrasonic vibration or other methods. They allow the dose to be inhaled at an appropriate rate and particle size, which ensure deposition of the preparation in the lungs. Metered-dose nebulizers are devices that convert liquids into aerosols by high-pressure gases, ultrasonic vibration or other methods. The volume of liquid to be nebulized is metered so that the aerosol dose can be inhaled with one breath.

(C) Pressurized Metered-Dose Preparations for inhalation

Pressurized inhalations are pressurized metered-dose preparations for inhalation. They are solutions, suspensions or emulsions supplied in special containers equipped with a metering valve and which are held under pressure with suitable propellants or suitable mixtures of liquefied propellants, which can act also as solvents. Suitable co-solvents, solubilizers and stabilizers may be added.

The formulation of the inhalation and the components of the delivery device (that is the pressurized container with its integral metering valve and the actuator) should be designed and, where appropriate, the particle size of the active ingredient should be controlled so that, when the pressurized inhalation is used in accordance with the manufacturer's recommendations, an adequate proportion of the active ingredient is made available for inhalation. A proportion of the active ingredient is deposited on the inner surface of the actuator; the amount available for inhalation is therefore less than the amount released by actuation of the valve. Pressurized inhalations should be manufactured in conditions designed to minimize microbial and particulate contamination.

2. Powders for Inhalation

Powders for inhalation are presented as single-dose powders or multi-dose powders. To facilitate their use, active substances may be combined with a suitable carrier. They are generally administered by dry-powder inhalers. In pre-metered systems, the inhaler is loaded with powders pre-dispensed in capsules or other suitable pharmaceutical forms. For devices using a powder reservoir, the dose is created by a metering mechanism within the inhaler.

The delivered dose is the dose delivered from the inhaler. For some preparations, the dose has been established as a metered dose or as a predispensed dose. The metered dose is determined by adding the amount deposited within the device to the delivered dose. It may also be determined directly.

Methods of Preparation

Some inhalations consist of one or more volatile oils and these oils are immiscible in aqueous vehicle hence for their uniform distribution in aqueous phase an adsorbent of diffusible nature is required e.g. Magnesium carbonate. It subdivides the oil sufficiently to ensure its uniform dispersion on shaking.

Volatile oils are triturated with adsorbents to breakdown oils into fine globules. When such inhalation (dispersion) is added to the hot water, a free vaporization of volatile oil takes place.

If the quantity of adsorbent is not mentioned in the formula then 1 g of light magnesium carbonate can be added for 2 ml of volatile oil and 2 g of volatile substances respectively.

Therapeutic Uses

Menthol-Eucalptus oil Inhalation BPC (Aqueous Inhalation) is used in the treatment of bronchitis and also acts as antiseptic, counter-irritant; therefore this inhalation is used for the relief of nasal congestion. Benzoin Inhalation BP is used as expectorant and anti-inflammatory agent for the treatment of throat and bronchial inflammation. Menthol inhalation can be used as anti-pruritic agent for treatment of nasal decongestion, headache and neuralgia.

Dose

The recommended dose of Benzoin Inhalation BP and Menthol and Benzoin Inhalation BP is 2 ml.

Storage Conditions

Higher temperature causes the volatilization of volatile oil/substances so inhalations should be stored in a cool place. Pressurized inhalations are supplied in suitable containers fitted with an appropriate metering valve that forms an integral part of the container. Metal containers comply with the relevant requirements of British Standard 3914: Part 1:1974 (non-returnable metal containers up to 1400 cm^3 and 85 mm diameter). The containers are usually supplied with an appropriate actuator.

Specific Labeling Requirement

The label on the container of inhalations should state (1) the names and concentrations of the active ingredients, (2) that the inhalation is not to be taken by mouth, (3) the date after which the inhalation is not intended to be used, and (4) the conditions under which the inhalation should be stored.

The label on the container of powders for inhalation should state (1) the date after which the powder for inhalation is not intended to be used, (2) the conditions under which the powder for inhalation should be stored. Where the powder for inhalation is supplied in a capsule, the label also states, (3) the quantity of the active ingredient contained in each capsule, and (4) that the capsules are intended for use in an inhaler and are not to be swallowed.

For metered-dose preparations the label states: the delivered dose, except for preparations for which the dose has been established as a metered-dose or as a predispensed-dose, where applicable, the number of deliveries from the inhaler to provide the minimum recommended dose, the number of deliveries per inhaler. The label states, where applicable, the name of any added antimicrobial preservative.

The label of pressurized inhalation states (1) the name of the active ingredient or ingredients, (2) the amount of active ingredient or ingredients delivered by each actuation of the valve and the number of deliveries available from the container, (3) the instructions for using the pressurized inhalation, (4) the date after which the pressurized inhalation is not intended to be used, (5) the conditions under which the pressurized inhalation should be stored, and (6) any special precautions associated with the use of the pressurized inhalation.

The label of solutions for nebulization should state (1) the date after which the solution for nebulization is not intended to be used, and (2) the conditions under which the solution for nebulization should be stored.

In addition, it should contain auxiliary label like, 'FOR EXTERNAL USE ONLY' or 'FOR NASAL USE ONLY', 'QUANTITY REQUIRED TO BE ADDED IN THE HOT WATER', 'STORE IN A COOL PLACE'.

Examples of Some Inhalations

1. Benzoin Inhalation BP

Benzoin Inhalation BP is an inhalation vapor solution. It is an extemporaneous preparation. In Benzoin Inhalation BP the content of total balsamic acids should not less than 3% w/v, calculated as cinnamic acid ($C_9H_8O_2$) and the total solids are 9 to 12% w/v when determined by drying at 105°C for 4 hours. The label of benzoin inhalation should indicate the pharmaceutical form as 'inhalation vapor'.

Composition	Method of Preparation
Sumatra benzoin crushed- 100 g Prepared storax of commerce- 50 g Ethanol (96%) q.s.- 1000 ml	Macerate the crushed sumatra benzoin and the prepared storax with 750 ml of ethanol (96%) for 24 hours. Filter and pass sufficient ethanol (96%) through the filter to produce 1000 ml. **Note-** In preparation of Benzoin Inhalation BP, ethanol (96%) may be replaced by industrial methylated spirit.

Label

<table>
<tr><td colspan="3" align="center">BENZOIN INHALATION BP
(50 ml)</td></tr>
<tr>
<td>Composition:

Each 50 ml contains,

Sumatra benzoin crushed- 5 g

Prepared storax of commerce- 2.5 g

Ethanol (96%) q.s.- 50 ml

Dose: As directed by physician.

Storage: Store in a tightly closed container in a cool place.</td>
<td align="center">MESALICYL

(Inhalation)

(Used in chronic bronchitis, pharyngitis and laryngitis)

PROTECT FROM SUN LIGHT</td>
<td>Mfg. Lic. No.- 5K/2010

Batch No.- AB 263

Mfg. Date- Apr. 2011

Exp. Date- Mar. 2012

M.R.P.- Rs. 28.00

(Inclusive of all taxes)

Mfd. By: YAVI PHARMA KANPUR ROAD, LUCKNOW UP- 226001</td>
</tr>
</table>

2. Menthol and Benzoin Inhalation BP

Menthol and Benzoin Inhalation BP is an inhalation vapor solution. It is an extemporaneous preparation. The content of total balsamic acids should not be less than 2.8% w/v, calculated as cinnamic acid, $(C_9H_8O_2)$ and the total solids should be 9 to 12% w/v when determined by drying at 105°C for 4 hours. The label indicates the pharmaceutical form as 'inhalation vapor'.

Composition	Method of Preparation
Race menthol or Levo menthol- 20 g Benzoin inhalation q.s.- 1000 ml	Dissolve the required quantity of Race-menthol or the Levo-menthol in a portion of the benzoin inhalation then add sufficient benzoin inhalation to produce 1000 ml and mix.

Label

<table>
<tr><td colspan="3" align="center">MENTHOL AND BENZOIN INHALATION BP
(50 ml)</td></tr>
<tr>
<td>Composition:
Each 50 ml contains,
Race menthol or Levo-menthol- 1 g
Benzoin Inhalation q.s.- 50 ml
Dose: As directed by physician
Storage: Store in a tightly closed container in a cool place.</td>
<td align="center">BENZOMENTH
(Inhalation)
(Used in chronic bronchitis)

PROTECT FROM SUN LIGHT</td>
<td>Mfg. Lic. No.- 4Z/2010
Batch No.- GH 142
Mfg. Date- July 2011
Exp. Date- June 2012
M.R.P.- Rs. 25.00
(Inclusive of all taxes)
Mfd. By: YAVI PHARMA KANPUR ROAD, LUCKNOW UP- 226001</td>
</tr>
</table>

3. Salbutamol Nebulizer Solution BP

Salbutamol Nebulizer Solution BP is a solution of salbutamol sulphate in water for injection. The content of salbutamol, ($C_{13}H_{21}NO_3$) is 95% to 105% of the stated amount. The pH of solution is 3 to 5. The label states the quantity of active ingredient in terms of the equivalent amount of salbutamol.

Composition	Method of Preparation
Salbutamol sulphate- 0.5 g Water for injection- 100 ml	Dissolve the required quantity of salbutamol sulphate in water for injection and make up the volume 100 ml.

Label

<table>
<tr><td colspan="3" align="center">SALBUTAMOL NEBULISER SOLUTION BP
(50 ml)</td></tr>
<tr>
<td>Composition:
Each 50 ml contains,
Salbutamol sulphate- 0.25 g
Water for injection q.s.- 50 ml
Dose: As directed by physician
Storage: Store in a tightly closed container in a cool place.</td>
<td align="center">SALBUTA-NEB
(Inhalation)
(Used in acute asthma)

PROTECT FROM SUN LIGHT</td>
<td>Mfg. Lic. No.- 2P/2010
Batch No.- CN 142
Mfg. Date- Aug. 2011
Exp. Date- July 2013
M.R.P.- Rs. 35.00
(Inclusive of all taxes)
Mfd. By: YAVI PHARMA KANPUR ROAD, LUCKNOW UP- 226001</td>
</tr>
</table>

4. Sodium Cromoglicate Powder for Inhalation

Sodium cromoglicate powder for inhalation consists of hard gelatin capsules containing either sodium cromoglicate appropriately treated or sodium cromoglicate admixed with an approximately equal amount of lactose. The content of sodium cromoglicate, $(C_{23}H_{14}Na_2O_{11})$ is 20.0 to 24.4 mg per capsule.

The label should state (1) that each capsule contains 20 mg of sodium cromoglicate, (2) that the capsules are intended for use in an inhaler and are not to be swallowed, and (3) that the capsules contain lactose, where applicable.

Composition	Method of Preparation
Sodium cromoglicate- 0.02 g Lactose- 0.02 g	Make a powder of sodium cromoglicate to a suitable fineness and mix the required quantity of lactose.

Label

SODIUM CROMOGLICATE POWDER FOR INHALATION (50 Capsules)		
Composition: Each capsule contains, Sodium cromoglicate- 0.02 g Lactose- 0.02 g **Dose:** As directed by physician. **Storage:** Store in a tightly closed container at a temperature not exceeding 30°C.	**CROMAL** (Inhalation powder) (Used as antiasthmatic) **PROTECT FROM MOISTURE** **DO NOT SWALLOW**	**Mfg. Lic. No.-** 2T/2010 **Batch No.-** CM 142 **Mfg. Date-** June 2011 **Exp. Date-** May 2013 **M.R.P.-** Rs. 105.00 (Inclusive of all taxes) **Mfd. By:** YAVI PHARMA KANPUR ROAD, LUCKNOW UP- 226001

5. Salbutamol Pressurized Inhalation BP

Salbutamol Pressurized Inhalation BP is a suspension of either salbutamol or salbutamol sulphate in a suitable liquid in a suitable pressurized container. The content of salbutamol $(C_{13}H_{21}NO_3)$ is 80% to 120% of the amount stated to be delivered by actuation of the valve. The label on the container states (1) whether the preparation contains salbutamol or salbutamol sulphate, (2) that the preparation does not contain, where applicable, and (3) when the active ingredient is salbutamol sulphate, the quantity is stated in terms of the equivalent amount of salbutamol.

Composition	Method of Preparation
Salbutamol sulphate- 0.02 g Propellant- q.s.	Suspend the required quantity of salbutamol sulphate in sufficient quantity of non-chlorofluorocarbon (CFCs) propellant.

Label

<table>
<tr><td colspan="3" align="center">SALBUTAMOL PRESSURISED INHALATION BP

(200 Metered Dose)</td></tr>
<tr>
<td>Composition:

Each metered dose contains,

Salbutamol sulphate- 100 mcg

Propellant- q.s.

Dose: As directed by physician.

Storage: Store in a pressurized container in a cool place.</td>
<td align="center">SALMOL

(Inhalation)

(Used as antiasthmatic)

PROTECT FROM SUN LIGHT

SHAKE WELL BEFORE USE</td>
<td>Mfg. Lic. No.- 2H/2010

Batch No.- SK 142

Mfg. Date- Sep. 2011

Exp. Date- Aug. 2013

M.R.P.- Rs. 95.00

(Inclusive of all taxes)

Mfd. By: YAVI PHARMA KANPUR ROAD, LUCKNOW UP- 226001</td>
</tr>
</table>

6. Beclomethasone Pressurized Inhalation BP

Beclomethasone Pressurized Inhalation BP is a solution or suspension of anhydrous beclomethasone dipropionate in a suitable liquid in a suitable pressurized container. The content of beclomethasone dipropionate, $(C_{28}H_{37}ClO_7)$ is 80% to 120% of the amount stated to be delivered by actuation of the valve.

Composition	Method of Preparation
Beclomethasone dipropionate- 0.02 g Propellant- q.s.	Suspend the required quantity of beclomethasone dipropionate in sufficient quantity of propellant.

Label

BECLOMETHASONE PRESSURISED INHALATION BP (200 Metered Dose)		
Composition: Each metered dose contains, Beclomethasone dipropionate - 100 mcg Propellant- q.s. **Dose:** As directed by physician. **Storage:** Store in a pressurized container in a cool place.	**BECLOMETH** (Inhalation) (Used as antiasthmatic) **PROTECT FROM SUN LIGHT** **SHAKE WELL BEFORE USE**	**Mfg. Lic. No.-** 3U/2010 **Batch No.-** MN 023 **Mfg. Date-** May 2011 **Exp. Date-** Apr. 2013 **M.R.P.-** Rs. 78.00 (Inclusive of all taxes) **Mfd. By:** YAVI PHARMA KANPUR ROAD, LUCKNOW UP- 226001

Marketed preparations

Active Ingredient(s)	Marketed Preparation (Manufacturer)
Salbutamol	**ASTHALIN** (CIPLA), **DERIHALER** (GERMAN REMEDIES), **DUOLIN** (CIPLA), **RESPISOL** (ALCHEMIST), **VENTORLIN** (GLAXO-SMITHKLINE)
Beclomethasone	**BECLATE-200** (CIPLA), **BECORIDE INHALER** (GLAXO-SMITHKLINE)
Budesonide	**BUDANASE AQ** (PROTEC), **BUDVENT INHALER** (KRESP), **BUDEZ** (NATCO), **PULMICORT** (ASTRA ZENECA)
Formoterol	**DUOVA** (CIPLA), **FORATEC INHALER** (CIPLA)
Fluticasone	**FLOHALE** (CIPLA)
Sodium cromoglycate	**IFIRAL** (UNIQUE)
Salmeterol	**VENT SF** (MERCK), **AZROL** (NATCO PHARMA), **SALMETER** (DR. REDDY'S LAB), **SEROBID** (CIPLA)

EXERCISE - 19

Object

To prepare and submit 50 ml Benzoin Inhalation BP.

Theory

Inhalations are solutions or suspensions of volatile substances administered by nasal or oral respiratory route in the form of vapor. Inhalations are administered either for their local action on the bronchial tree or for their systemic effects through absorption from lungs. Benzoin is an oleo-resin obtained from stems of *Storax benzoin*. Prepared storax is a balsam obtained from the trunk of *Liquidamber orientalis*.

Formula

Ingredients	Quantity Required
Sumatra benzoin crushed	100 g
Prepared storax	50 g
Ethanol (96%) q.s. to	1000 ml

Apparatus

Glass beaker, measuring cylinder and volumetric pipette.

Procedure

Benzoin Inhalation BP is prepared by maceration of crushed benzoin and prepared storax with alcohol (96%). Crush the benzoin into small pieces. Accurately weigh benzoin and prepared storax and macerate them with ¾ᵗʰ quantity of alcohol (96%) in a closed vessel for 24 hours. After 24 hours, filter and pass the sufficient amount of alcohol (96%) through filter to produce final volume and mix well.

Category

Expectorant and soothing by steam inhalation in acute laryngitis.

Dose

5 to 10 ml.

Therapeutic use

Benzoin Inhalation BP is used as expectorant and anti-inflammatory agent for the treatment of throat and bronchial inflammation.

Storage

Benzoin Inhalation BP should be stored in amber colored, narrow mouth glass bottle and close it tightly with plastic screw cap. Higher temperature leads to the volatilization of volatile substances hence it should be stored in cool place.

Label

'FOR EXTERNAL USE ONLY' or 'FOR NASAL USE ONLY', 'SHAKE WELL BEFORE USE'.

Note: Inhalants differ from inhalation in that the former are drugs or combination of drugs which can be carried out by an air current into nasal passage to exert their effects by virtue of their high vapor pressure.

Specimen Label

The specimen label for Benzoin Inhalation BP is given as:

BENZOIN INHALATION BP (50 ml)		
Composition: Each 50 ml contains, Sumatra benzoin- 5 g Prepared storax- 2.5 g Ethanol (96%) q.s.- 50 ml **Dose:** 5 to 10 ml **Storage:** Store in well closed, narrow mouthed, amber colored glass bottle in cool place and close it tightly with plastic screw cap.	**BENZ INHALATION** (Inhalation) **Expectorant** (Used as expectorant and anti-inflammatory agent) **FOR EXTERNAL USE ONLY** **SHAKE WELL BEFORE USE**	**Mfg. Lic. No.-** 8J/2010 **Batch No.-** JM 0512 **Mfg. Date-** May 2011 **Exp. Date-** Apr. 2012 **M.R.P.-** Rs. 45.00 (Inclusive of all taxes) **Mfd. By:** YAVI PHARMA KANPUR ROAD, LUCKNOW UP- 226001

CHAPTER 12

TINCTURES AND EXTRACTS

Extracts are preparations of liquid (liquid extracts and tinctures), semi-solid (soft extracts) or solid (dry extracts) consistency, obtained from herbal drugs or animal matters, which are usually in a dry state.

Liquid extracts are liquid preparations of which, in general, 1 part by mass or volume is equivalent to 1 part by mass of the dried herbal drug or animal matter. These preparations are adjusted, if necessary, so that they satisfy the requirements for content of solvent, and, where applicable, for constituents.

Tinctures are liquid preparations which are usually obtained using either 1 part of herbal drug or animal matter and 10 parts of extraction solvent or 1 part of herbal drug or animal matter and 5 parts of extraction solvent.

A 'tincture' contains one drug while compound tincture contains more than one vegetable or animal drug. Soft extracts are semisolid preparations obtained by evaporation or partial evaporation of the solvent used for extraction. Dry extracts are solid preparations obtained by evaporation of the solvent used for their production. Dry extracts usually have a loss on drying or a water content of not greater than 5% w/w. It should be stored in an airtight container, protected from light.

A tincture is an alcohol-based derivative of a fresh herb or other natural plant material, used primarily as an alternative medicine or dietary supplement. Tincture may be a solution of a non-volatile substance (e.g. of iodine, mercurochrome). To qualify as a tincture, the alcoholic extract is to have an ethanol percentage of at least 40-60% (sometimes a 90% pure liquid may be achieved). Chemically, a tincture is a solution that has alcohol as the solvent. The alcohol, glycerin or vinegar used in a tincture added stability to the concentrated chemicals found in the herbs. Tinctures are usually clear. A slight sediment may form on standing which is acceptable as long as the composition of the tincture is not changed significantly. Official tinctures vary greatly in their methods of preparation, active ingredients, alcoholic content and the intended use.

Some examples of tinctures that were formerly common in medicine include- Tincture of *Cannabis sativa*, tincture of benzoin, tincture of cantharides, tincture of ferric citro-

141

chloride, tincture of green soap, tincture of guaiac, tincture of iodine, tincture of opium, camphorated opium tincture and tincture of pennyroyal.

Methods of Preparation

Extracts are prepared by suitable methods using ethanol or other suitable solvents. Different batches of the herbal drug or animal matter may be blended prior to extraction. The herbal drug or animal matter to be extracted may undergo a preliminary treatment, for example, inactivation of enzymes, grinding or defatting. In addition, unwanted matter may be removed after extraction.

Herbal drugs, animal matters and organic solvents used for the preparation of extracts comply with any relevant monograph of the Pharmacopoeia. For soft and dry extracts recovered or recycled solvent may be used, but the recovery procedures should be controlled and monitored to ensure that solvents meet appropriate standards before reuse or admixture with other approved materials. Water used for the preparation of extracts is of suitable quality. Except for the test for bacterial endotoxins, water complying with the monograph of purified water is suitable. Potable water may be suitable if it complies with a defined specification that allows the consistent production of a suitable extract.

Where applicable, concentration to the intended consistency is carried out using suitable methods, usually under reduced pressure, and at a temperature at which deterioration of the constituents is reduced to a minimum. Essential oils that have been separated during processing may be restored to the extracts at an appropriate stage in the manufacturing process. Suitable excipients may be added at various stages of the manufacturing process, for example, to improve technological qualities such as homogeneity or consistency. Suitable stabilizers and antimicrobial preservatives may also be added.

Liquid extracts are prepared by using ethanol of suitable concentration or water to extract the herbal drug or animal matter, or by dissolving a soft or dry extract (which has been produced using the same strength of extraction solvent as is used in preparing the liquid extract by direct extraction) of the herbal drug or animal matter in either ethanol of suitable concentration or water. Liquid extracts may be filtered, if necessary. A slight sediment may form on standing, which is acceptable as long as the composition of the liquid extract is not changed significantly.

During the general procedure of preparation of tinctures, herbs are put in a jar and pure ethanol is added at 40°C. The jar is left to stand for 2-3 weeks with occasional shaking. With most of the tinctures 1 part water at 5 parts ethanol is used but depending on the herb, to make a more precise tincture, 1 part herbs with 2-10 parts of water-ethanol mixture can be used.

Commercially tinctures are prepared by maceration or percolation method using only ethanol of a suitable concentration for extraction of the herbal drug or animal matter, or by dissolving a soft or dry extract (which has been produced using the same strength of extraction solvent as is used in preparing the tincture by direct extraction) of the herbal drug or animal matter in ethanol of a suitable concentration. Tinctures are filtered, if necessary.

Production by Maceration (Process M)

Unless otherwise prescribed, reduce the herbal drug or animal matter to be extracted to pieces of suitable size, mix thoroughly with the prescribed extraction solvent and allow to stand in a closed container for an appropriate time. The residue is separated from the extraction solvent and, if necessary, pressed out. In the latter case, the two liquids obtained are combined. For the maceration, place the solid materials with the whole of the menstruum in a closed vessel and allow to stand for 7 days, shaking occasionally. Strain, press the marc and mix the liquids obtained. Clarify by subsidence or filtration.

In process M [USP], macerate the drug with 750 ml of the prescribed solvent or solvent mixture in a container that can be closed, and put in a warm place. Agitate it frequently during three days or until the soluble matter is dissolved. Transfer the mixture to a filter, and when most of the liquid has drained away, wash the residue on the filter with a sufficient quantity of the prescribed solvent or solvent mixture, combining the filters, to produce 1000 ml of tincture and mix.

Production by Percolation (Process P)

If necessary, reduce the herbal drug or animal matter to be extracted to pieces of suitable size. Mix thoroughly with a portion of the prescribed extraction solvent and allow to stand for an appropriate time. Transfer to a percolator and allow the percolate to flow at room temperature slowly making sure that the herbal drug or animal matter to be extracted is always covered with the remaining extraction solvent. The residue may be pressed out and the expressed liquid combined with the percolate.

For percolation, moisten the solid materials with a sufficient quantity of the menstruum, allow to stand for 4 hours in a well-closed vessel, pack in a percolator and add sufficient of the menstruum to saturate the materials. When the liquid begins to drop from the percolator, close the outlet, add sufficient of the menstruum to leave a layer above the drug and allow to macerate for 24 hours. Allow percolation to proceed slowly until the percolate measures about three-quarters of the required volume. Press the marc, mix the expressed liquid with the percolate and add sufficient of the menstruum to produce the required volume. Clarify by subsidence or filtration.

Continuous extraction of a drug for the purpose of an assay consists of percolating the drug with the solvent stated in the monograph at a temperature approximately that of the boiling point of the solvent. The apparatus should permit the uniform percolation of the drug and the regular flow of the vapor of the solvent around the percolator.

In process P [USP], carefully mix the ground drug or mixture of drugs with a sufficient quantity of the prescribed solvent or solvent mixture to render it evenly and distinctly damp, allow it to stand for 15 minutes. Transfer it to a suitable percolator, and pack the drug firmly. Pour on enough of the prescribed solvent or solvent mixture to saturate the drug, cover the top of the percolator, and when the liquid is about to drip from the percolator, close the lower orifice an allow the drug to macerate for 24 hours or for the time specified in the monograph. If no assay is directed, allow the percolation to proceed slowly or at the specified rate, gradually adding sufficient solvent or solvent mixture to produce 1000 ml of tincture, and mix.

The Choice of Extraction Method

The choice of extraction method depends primarily on the physical properties of the basic material and its particle size. If this material is a coarse, rigid powder, beds of high permeability will form and percolation can be adopted. The expense of finer grinding is avoided, and the subsequent separation of solids and liquid is facilitated. The process can be conducted in such a way that a concentrated product is obtained. Other materials, such as fine powders or compressible animal tissues, will not form permeable beds, and the alternative method must be adopted. Some compensation for the difficulties of separation and the dilution of the extract during washing may be found in a more rapid and more complete extraction, due to the use of finer powders, the intimate contact between solids and liquid, and the absence of channeling. The use of pressure extends the application of percolation to materials which form beds of low permeability. Alternatively, permeability may be increased by grinding the solids with a supporting material such as glass wool.

The Choice of Solvent

The ideal solvent is cheap, nontoxic, and noninflammable. It is highly selective, dissolving only the wanted constituents of the solid. It should have a low viscosity, allowing easy movement through a bed of solids, and, if the resulting solution is to be concentrated by evaporation, a high vapor pressure. These factors greatly limit the number of solvents of commercial value. Water and alcohol, and mixtures of the two, are widely used. Both, however, are nonselective, leaching varying proportions of gums, mucilages, and other unwanted components. Most of the tinctures and liquid extracts used in pharmacy are simple, impure extracts made with water or mixtures of water and alcohol. Acidified or alkaline mixtures of water and alcohol are used to extract insulin from minced pancreas. A more selective extraction is given by petroleum solvents and benzene and related solvents. In the preparation of many pure alkaloids, the powdered material is moistened with an alkaline solution, packed into a bed, and leached with petroleum. Subsequent purification by fractional crystallization is facilitated by the absence of gums. Acetone and chlorinated hydrocarbons also find applications in leaching. In some cases, specific properties of the wanted constituents may suggest a particular solvent. Eugenol, for example, can be readily extracted from cloves with a solution of potassium hydroxide. Care must be given to the selection of solvents, because they may be subject to regulatory control due to their toxicity or impact on the environment.

Therapeutic Uses

Medicated tinctures taken orally include Camphorated Tincture of Opium USP (Paregoric) and Opium Tincture USP (Laudanum) but later is much more potent than former. Internally tinctures are used as cardiotonics (e.g. Digitalis tincture), as anticholinergics (e.g. Belladonna tincture) and as emetics (e.g. Ipecacuanha tincture). Some tinctures are used as flavoring agents (e.g. Orange Tincture IP or Sweet Orange Peel Tincture USP).

Dose

Most tincture recipes require one tablespoon to be consumed at mealtime at least once a day. The ultimate point of a tincture is not to cause intoxication, but to provide the strongest possible concentration of an herb's healing essences. The dose of tincture is usually 15 to 30 ml.

Storage Conditions

Because of the alcoholic content, tinctures must be tightly stoppered and not exposed to excessive temperatures. Also, because many of the constituents found in tinctures undergo a photochemical change upon exposure to light, tinctures must be stored in light resistant containers and protected from sunlight. Storage in a cool place will also minimize the evaporation of alcohol. The tinctures whose active ingredients alter with time (e.g. Aconite tincture, Belladonna tincture and Hyoscyamous tincture) should be discarded after one year.

Specific Labeling Requirement

The label should state the ethanol content in % v/v in the final tincture, for tinctures other than standardized and quantified tinctures, the ratio of starting material to extraction liquid or of starting material to final tincture.

Examples of Some Tinctures

1. Tincture of Benzoin USP

Tincture of Benzoin USP is a pungent solution of benzoin resin in alcohol. Tincture of Benzoin USP has two main medical uses, as a treatment for damaged skin, and as an inhalant. It is often applied to skin before applying tape or other adhesive bandages. To some degree, it protects the skin from allergy to the adhesive in the tape or bandage, but mostly it makes the tape or bandages adhere much longer. It is also used by athletes for its reputation of toughening skin exposed to the tincture. It can be applied to minor cuts as a styptic and antiseptic (an effect of both the benzoin and its alcohol solvent). It is also used as an oral mucosal protectant, for recurring canker sores (a small ulcer of mouth or lips), fever blisters. It can also be inhaled in steam as a treatment for various conditions including bronchitis and colds.

Composition	Method of Preparation
Benzoin (crushed)- 20 g Alcohol (95%) q.s.- 100 ml	Macerate the benzoin (crushed) in 80 ml of alcohol for 1 hour with frequent agitation, filter and pass sufficient alcohol through the filter to make the volume 100 ml.

Label

TINCTURE OF BENZOIN USP **(50 ml)**		
Composition: Each 50 ml contains, Benzoin (crushed)- 10 g Alcohol (95%) q.s.- 50 ml **Dose:** 1-2 ml **Storage:** Store in a tightly closed light-resistant container in a cool place.	**BENZOTIN** (Tincture) (Used for inhalation in bronchitis) **PROTECT FROM SUN LIGHT** **FOR EXTERNAL USE ONLY**	**Mfg. Lic. No.-** 2J/2010 **Batch No.-** BN 713 **Mfg. Date-** Apr. 2011 **Exp. Date-** Mar. 2012 **M.R.P.-** Rs. 20.00 (Inclusive of all taxes) **Mfd. By:** YAVI PHARMA KANPUR ROAD, LUCKNOW UP- 226001

2. Belladonna Tincture BP; USP

Belladonna Tincture BP	Belladonna Tincture USP
It is an extemporaneous preparation. The content of alkaloids is 0.028 to 0.032% w/v, calculated as hyoscyamine, and ethanol content is 64 to 69% v/v.	Alcohol content is between 65-70%. It yields, from each 100 ml, not less than 27 mg and not more than 33 mg of the alkaloids of belladonna leaf.
Composition: Belladonna herb (moderately coarse powder)- 100 g Ethanol (70%) q.s.- 1000 ml	**Composition:** Belladonna leaf (moderately coarse powder)- 100 g Ethanol (70%) q.s.- 1000 ml
Method of preparation: About 900 ml of a tincture is prepared by percolation method (Process P). Finally adjust the volume of tincture with ethanol (70%) to contain 0.03% w/v of alkaloids.	**Method of preparation:** It is prepared by Process M using a mixture of 3 volumes of alcohol and 1 volume of water as the menstruum. Finally adjust the volume of tincture to contain in each 100 ml, 30 mg of the alkaloids of belladonna leaf.

Label

BELLADONNA TINCTURE BP		
(50 ml)		
Composition: Each 50 ml contains, Belladonna herb- 5 g Ethanol (70%) q.s.- 50 ml **Dose:** As directed by physician **Storage:** Store in tight, light-resistant containers, and exposure to direct sunlight and excessive heat should be avoided.	**DONNA-TINCTURE** (Tincture) (Used as a sedative and antispasmodic) **PROTECT FROM SUN LIGHT** **NOT FOR INJECTION**	**Mfg. Lic. No.-** 4H/2010 **Batch No.-** BN 0115 **Mfg. Date-** Feb. 2011 **Exp. Date-** Jan. 2012 **M.R.P.-** Rs. 20.00 (Inclusive of all taxes) **Mfd. By:** YAVI PHARMA KANPUR ROAD, LUCKNOW UP- 226001

3. Compound Benzoin Tincture IP; BP

Compound Benzoin Tincture (Friar's Balsam) IP	Compound Benzoin Tincture BP
The ethanol content is 70 to 77% v/v. It has relative density 0.870 to 0.885 and dry residue not less than 13.5% w/v, determined on 1 ml by drying in an oven at 105°C for 4 hours. **Composition:** Benzoin (moderately coarse powder)- 100 g Prepared storax- 75 g Tolu balsam- 25 g Aloes (moderately coarse powder)- 20 g Ethanol (90%) q.s.- 1000 ml **Method of preparation:** Macerate the benzoin, prepared storax, Tolu balsam and aloes with 800 ml of ethanol (90%) in a closed vessel for not less than 48 hours, shaking occasionally, filter and pass sufficient ethanol (90%) through the filter to produce 1000 ml.	It is an extemporaneous preparation. The content of total balsamic acids should not be less than 4.5% w/v, calculated as cinnamic acid, $(C_9H_8O_2)$. The ethanol content is 70 to 76% v/v. It has relative density 0.880 to 0.910 and dry residue 15 to 19% w/v. **Composition:** Barbados Aloes / Cape Aloes- 20 g Prepared storax of commerce- 100 g Sumatra Benzoin crushed- 100 g Ethanol (90%) q.s.- 1000 ml **Method of preparation:** Macerate the Barbados aloes or Cape aloes, the prepared storax and the Sumatra Benzoin with 800 ml of ethanol (90%) in a closed vessel for not less than 2 days, shaking occasionally, filter and pass sufficient ethanol (90%) through the filter to produce 1000 ml.

Label

COMPOUND BENZOIN TINCTURE (FRIAR'S BALSAM) IP (50 ml)		
Composition: Each 50 ml contains, Benzoin- 5 g Prepared storax- 3.75 g Tolu balsam- 1.25 g Aloes- 1 g Ethanol (90%) q.s.- 50 ml **Dose:** 2-4 ml **Storage:** Store in tight, light-resistant container.	**COMBENZ** (Tincture) (Used in chronic bronchitis) **PROTECT FROM SUN LIGHT** **SHAKE WELL BEFORE USE**	**Mfg. Lic. No.-** 2W/2010 **Batch No.-** CK 0153 **Mfg. Date-** Feb. 2011 **Exp. Date-** Jan. 2012 **M.R.P.-** Rs. 22.00 (Inclusive of all taxes) **Mfd. By:** YAVI PHARMA KANPUR ROAD, LUCKNOW UP- 226001

4. Compound Cardamom Tincture USP

The alcohol content is between 43% and 47% v/v.

Composition	Method of Preparation
Cardamom seed (moderately coarse powder)- 20 g Cinnamon (fine powder)- 25 g Caraway (moderately coarse powder)- 12 g Diluted alcohol q.s.- 1000 ml	Macerate the mixed powders in 750 ml of a mixture of 50 ml of glycerin and 950 ml of diluted alcohol, and complete the preparation by using first the remainder of the mixture of diluted alcohol and glycerin prepared as directed above, followed by diluted alcohol.

Label

COMPOUND CARDAMOM TINCTURE USP (50 ml)		
Composition: Each 50 ml contains, Cardamom seed- 1 g Cinnamon- 1.25 g Caraway- 0.6 g Diluted alcohol q.s.- 50 ml **Dose:** 2-4 ml **Storage:** Store in tight, light-resistant container, and avoid exposure to direct sunlight and excessive heat.	**COMCARDA** (Tincture) (Used as carminative) **PROTECT FROM SUN LIGHT** **SHAKE WELL BEFORE USE**	**Mfg. Lic. No.-** 5D/2010 **Batch No.-** CK 103 **Mfg. Date-** Aug. 2011 **Exp. Date-** July. 2012 **M.R.P.-** Rs. 28.00 (Inclusive of all taxes) **Mfd. By:** YAVI PHARMA KANPUR ROAD, LUCKNOW UP- 226001

5. Lemon Tincture USP

Composition	Method of Preparation
Lemon peel- 500 g Alcohol q.s.- 1000 ml	It is prepared from lemon peel which is outer yellow rind of the fresh, ripe fruit of *Citrus limon* (Family- Rutaceae). It is prepared by Process M. Macerate 500 g of the lemon peel in 900 ml of alcohol in a closed container and store in a warm place. Agitate the container frequently for 3 days or until the soluble matter is dissolved. Transfer the mixture to a filter, using talc as the filtering medium, and when most of the liquid has drained away, wash the residue on the filter with a sufficient amount of alcohol and combine the filtrates so that the preparation is brought to a final volume of 1000 ml.

Label

<table>
<tr><td colspan="3">LEMON TINCTURE USP
(50 ml)</td></tr>
<tr>
<td>Composition:
Each 50 ml contains,
Lemon peel- 25 g
Alcohol q.s.- 50 ml
Storage: Store in tight, light-resistant container at controlled room temperature, avoiding exposure to direct sunlight and to excessive heat.</td>
<td>LEM-TINCTURE
(Tincture)
(Used as a flavoring agent)

PROTECT FROM SUN LIGHT
SHAKE WELL BEFORE USE</td>
<td>Mfg. Lic. No.- 4H/2010
Batch No.- JK 021
Mfg. Date- Mar. 2011
Exp. Date- Feb. 2012
M.R.P.- Rs. 20.00
(Inclusive of all taxes)
Mfd. By: YAVI PHARMA KANPUR ROAD, LUCKNOW UP- 226001</td>
</tr>
</table>

6. Sweet Orange Peel Tincture USP

It is prepared from sweet orange peel which is the outer rind of the non-artificially colored, fresh, ripe fruit of *Citrus sinesis* (Family- Rutaceae). Alcohol content is between 62% and 72% v/v. The label should state the latin bionomial and the official name.

Composition	Method of Preparation
Sweet orange peel- 500 g Alcohol q.s.- 1000 ml	This tincture is prepared by Process M. Macerate 500 g of sweet orange peel in 900 ml of alcohol, and dilute the preparation with alcohol to make the product measure 1000 ml. Talc is used as a filtering medium.

Label

SWEET ORANGE PEEL TINCTURE USP (50 ml)		
Composition: Each 50 ml contains, Sweet orange peel - 25 g Alcohol q.s.- 50 ml **Storage:** Store in tight, light-resistant container, avoiding exposure to direct sunlight and to excessive heat.	**ORATIN** (Tincture) (Used as a flavoring agent) **PROTECT FROM SUN LIGHT** **SHAKE WELL BEFORE USE**	**Mfg. Lic. No.**-3R/2010 **Batch No.**- CK 032 **Mfg. Date**- Aug. 2011 **Exp. Date**- July 2012 **M.R.P.**- Rs. 19.00 (Inclusive of all taxes) **Mfd. By:** YAVI PHARMA KANPUR ROAD, LUCKNOW UP- 226001

7. Tolu Balsam Tincture USP

Alcohol content is between 77% and 83% v/v. The label should state the latin bionomial name and, following the official name, the part of the plant source from which it was derived.

Composition	Method of Preparation
Tolu balsam- 200 g Alcohol q.s.- 1000 ml	It is prepared from Tolu balsam obtained from *Myroxylon balsamum* (Family- Fabaceae). It is prepared by following Process M, using alcohol as the menstruum.

Label

TOLU BALSAM TINCTURE USP (50 ml)		
Composition: Each 50 ml contains, Tolu balsam- 200 g Alcohol q.s.- 1000 ml **Dose:** As directed by physician **Storage:** Store in tight, light-resistant container at controlled room temperature. Exposure to direct sunlight and excessive heat should be avoided.	**TOLUBAL** (Tincture) (Used as stimulant and expectorant) **PROTECT FROM SUN LIGHT** **SHAKE WELL BEFORE USE**	**Mfg. Lic. No.**- 4M/2010 **Batch No.**- SA 012 **Mfg. Date**- Sep. 2011 **Exp. Date**- Aug. 2012 **M.R.P.**- Rs. 22.00 (Inclusive of all taxes) **Mfd. By:** YAVI PHARMA KANPUR ROAD, LUCKNOW UP- 226001

8. Ginger Tincture USP

It contains not less than 0.10% of gingerols. The alcohol content should not be less than 90% and not more than 110%. It has specific gravity between 0.90 and 0.95.

Composition	Method of Preparation
Ginger- 200 g Mixture of alcohol and water (7:3) q.s.- 1000 ml	This tincture is prepared by the maceration process (Process M).

Label

<table>
<tr><td colspan="3" align="center">GINGER TINCTURE USP

(50 ml)</td></tr>
<tr>
<td>Composition:

Each 50 ml contains,

Ginger- 10 g

Alcohol and water (7:3) q.s.- 50 ml

Storage: Store in tight, light-resistant container at controlled room temperature. Exposure to direct sunlight and excessive heat should be avoided.</td>
<td align="center">GINTURE

(Tincture)

(Used as carminative and flavoring agent)

PROTECT FROM SUN LIGHT

SHAKE WELL BEFORE USE</td>
<td>Mfg. Lic. No.- 2G/2010

Batch No.- NM 297

Mfg. Date- Apr. 2011

Exp. Date- Mar. 2012

M.R.P.- Rs. 22.00

(Inclusive of all taxes)

Mfd. By: YAVI PHARMA KANPUR ROAD, LUCKNOW UP- 226001</td>
</tr>
</table>

9. Green Soap Tincture USP

Composition	Method of preparation
Green soap- 650 g Essential oil and alcohol- 316 ml Purified water q.s- 1000 ml	Mix the oil and alcohol, dissolve the green soap in this solution by stirring or by agitation, set the solution aside for 24 hours, filter through paper, and add purified water in a sufficient quantity to make volume 1000 ml. It has alcohol content between 28% and 32% v/v.

Label

<table>
<tr><td colspan="3" align="center">GREEN SOAP TINCTURE USP
(50 ml)</td></tr>
<tr>
<td>Composition:
Each 50 ml contains,
Green soap- 3.25 g
Essential oil and alcohol- 15.8 ml
Purified water q.s- 50 ml
Storage: Store in a tightly closed container.</td>
<td align="center">GREESOTIN
(Tincture)

PROTECT FROM SUN LIGHT
FOR EXTERNAL USE ONLY</td>
<td>Mfg. Lic. No.- 3F/2010
Batch No.- GH 156
Mfg. Date- Apr. 2011
Exp. Date- Mar. 2012
M.R.P.- Rs. 20.00
(Inclusive of all taxes)
Mfd. By: YAVI PHARMA KANPUR ROAD, LUCKNOW UP- 226001</td>
</tr>
</table>

10. Iodine Tincture USP

Iodine Tincture USP contains, in each 10 ml, iodine not less than 1.8 g and not more than 2.2 g and sodium iodide not less than 2.1 g and not more than 2.6 g. It has alcohol content between 44% and 50% v/v.

Composition	Method of Preparation
Iodine- 20 g Sodium iodide- 24 g Alcohol- 500 ml Purified water q.s.- 1000 ml	It may be prepared by dissolving required quantity of iodine and sodium iodide in 500 ml of alcohol and then adding purified water in a sufficient quantity to make the product measure 1000 ml.

Label

<table>
<tr><td colspan="3" align="center">IODINE TINCTURE USP
(50 ml)</td></tr>
<tr>
<td>Composition:
Each 50 ml contains,
Iodine- 1 g
Sodium iodide- 1.2 g
Alcohol- 25 ml
Purified water q.s.- 50 ml
Storage: Store in tight, light-resistant containers.</td>
<td align="center">IODIN-TINCTURE
(Tincture)
(Used as antiseptic)

PROTECT FROM SUN LIGHT
SHAKE WELL BEFORE USE</td>
<td>Mfg. Lic. No.- 2L/2010
Batch No.- SK 256
Mfg. Date- Apr. 2011
Exp. Date- Mar. 2012
M.R.P.- Rs. 23.00
(Inclusive of all taxes)
Mfd. By: YAVI PHARMA KANPUR ROAD, LUCKNOW UP- 226001</td>
</tr>
</table>

11. Strong Iodine Tincture USP

It contains, in each 100 ml, iodine not less than 6.8 g and not more than 7.5 g, and potassium iodide not less than 4.7 g and not more than 5.5 g. It has alcohol content between 82.5% and 88.5% v/v.

Composition	Method of Preparation
Iodine- 70 g Potassium iodide- 50 g Purified water- 50 ml Alcohol q.s.- 1000 ml	Dissolve potassium iodide (50 g) in 50 ml of purified water then add iodine (70 g), and agitate until solution is effected and then add alcohol to make the volume 1000 ml.

Label

STRONG IODINE TINCTURE USP (50 ml)		
Composition: Each 50 ml contains, Iodine- 3.5 g Potassium iodide- 2.5 g Purified water- 2.5 ml Alcohol q.s.- 50 ml **Storage:** Store in tight, light-resistant container.	**STRODINE** (Tincture) (Used as antiseptic) **PROTECT FROM SUN LIGHT** **FOR EXTERNAL USE ONLY**	**Mfg. Lic. No.-** 3L/2010 **Batch No.-** CM 012 **Mfg. Date-** Aug. 2011 **Exp. Date-** July. 2012 **M.R.P.-** Rs. 27.00 (Inclusive of all taxes) **Mfd. By:** YAVI PHARMA KANPUR ROAD, LUCKNOW UP- 226001

12. Opium Tincture USP

It contains, in each 10 ml, not less than 0.90 g and not more than 1.10 g of anhydrous morphine. It has alcohol content between 17% and 21% v/v.

Composition	Method of Preparation	Caution
Opium (sliced)- 100 g Alcohol- 188 ml Purified water q.s.- 1000 ml	It may be prepared by placing 100 g of granulated or sliced opium in a suitable vessel, add 500 ml of boiling water, and allow to stand, with frequent stirring, for 24 hours. Transfer the mixture to a percolator, allow it to drain, percolate with water as the menstruum to complete extraction, and evaporate the percolate to a volume of 400 ml. Boil actively for not less than 15 minutes, and allow to stand	Do not use powdered opium.

	overnight. Heat the mixture to 80°C then add 50 g of paraffin, and heat until the paraffin is melted. Shake the mixture thoroughly, and cool. Remove the paraffin, and filter the concentrate, washing the paraffin and the filter with the sufficient water to make the filtrate measure 750 ml. Add 188 ml of alcohol to the filtrate, mix. Dilute and mix the solution with a mixture of 1 volume of alcohol and 4 volumes of water to obtain a tincture containing 1 g of anhydrous morphine in each 100 ml.	

Label

OPIUM TINCTURE USP

(50 ml)

| **Composition:**
Each 50 ml contains,
Opium- 5 g
Alcohol- 9.4 ml
Purified water q.s.- 50 ml
Dose: 2-8 ml
Storage: Store in tight, light-resistant container. Exposure to direct sunlight and excessive heat should be avoided. | **OPI-TINCTURE**
(Tincture)
(Used as sedative and hypnotic)

PROTECT FROM SUN LIGHT
SHAKE WELL BEFORE USE | **Mfg. Lic. No.-** 2H/2010
Batch No.- AV 202
Mfg. Date- Apr. 2011
Exp. Date- Mar. 2012
M.R.P.- Rs. 30.00
(Inclusive of all taxes)
Mfd. By: YAVI PHARMA KANPUR ROAD, LUCKNOW UP- 226001 |

13. Vanilla Tincture USP

It has alcohol content between 38% and 42% v/v. The label should state the latin bionomial name and, following the official name, the part of the plant source from which it was derived.

Composition	Method of Preparation
Vanilla (powder)- 100 g Purified water- 200 ml Alcohol- 207 ml Sucrose- 200 g Diluted alcohol q.s.- 1000 ml	Add purified water to the powdered vanilla in a suitable covered container, and macerate for 12 hours, preferably in a warm place. Then add alcohol to the mixture, mix, and macerate for about 3 days. Transfer the mixture to a percolator containing sucrose, and drain. Pack the drug firmly and percolate slowly, using diluted alcohol as the menstruum.

Label

VANILLA TINCTURE USP (50 ml)		
Composition: Each 50 ml contains, Vanilla- 5 g Purified water- 10 ml Alcohol- 10.35 ml Sucrose- 10 g Diluted alcohol q.s.- 50 ml **Storage:** Store in tight, light-resistant container.	**VANILTURE** (Tincture) (Used as a flavoring agent) **PROTECT FROM SUN LIGHT** **SHAKE WELL BEFORE USE**	**Mfg. Lic. No.-** 1Q/2010 **Batch No.-** AY 253 **Mfg. Date-** Apr. 2011 **Exp. Date-** Mar. 2012 **M.R.P.-** Rs. 19.00 (Inclusive of all taxes) **Mfd. By:** YAVI PHARMA KANPUR ROAD, LUCKNOW UP- 226001

14. Benzethonium Chloride Tincture USP

It contains, in each 100 ml, not less than 190 mg and not more than 210 mg of benzethonium chloride. It has specific gravity between 0.868 and 0.876.

Composition	Method of Preparation
Bezethonium chloride- 2 g Alcohol- 685 ml Acetone- 10 ml Purified water q.s.- 1000 ml	Dissolve the benzethonium chloride in a mixture of alcohol and acetone then add sufficient purified water to make 1000 ml. It may be colored by the addition of any suitable color or combination of colors certified by the FDA for use in drugs.

Label

BENZETHONIUM CHLORIDE TINCTURE USP (50 ml)		
Composition: Each 50 ml contains, Bezethonium chloride- 0.1 g Alcohol- 34.25 ml Acetone- 0.5 ml Purified water q.s.- 1000 ml **Storage:** Store in tight, light-resistant container.	**BENZETH** (Tincture) **PROTECT FROM SUN LIGHT** **SHAKE WELL BEFORE USE**	**Mfg. Lic. No.-** 2N/2010 **Batch No.-** GH 472 **Mfg. Date-** Apr. 2011 **Exp. Date-** Mar. 2012 **M.R.P.-** Rs. 20.00 (Inclusive of all taxes) **Mfd. By:** YAVI PHARMA KANPUR ROAD, LUCKNOW UP- 226001

15. Belladonna Extract USP

Belladonna extract contains, in each 100 g, not less than 1.15 g and not more than 1.35 g of the alkaloids of belladonna leaf.

Pilular Belladonna Extract USP	Powdered Belladonna Extract USP
Composition:	**Composition:**
Belladonna leaf- 1000 g	Belladonna leaf- 1000 g
Alcohol and water (3:1) q.s.- 1000 ml	Alcohol q.s.- 1000 ml
Method of preparation: Prepare the extract by percolating 1000 g of belladonna leaf, using a mixture of 3 volumes of alcohol and 1 volume of water as the menstruum. Macerate the drug for 16 hours, and then percolate under reduced pressure and at a temperature not exceeding 60°C to a pilular consistency, and adjust the remaining extract, after assaying, by dilution with liquid glucose so that the finished extract will contain,1.25 g of the alkaloids of belladonna leaf in each 100 g.	**Method of preparation:** Prepare the extract by percolating 1000 g of belladonna leaf, using alcohol as the menstruum. Macerate the drug for 16 hours, and then percolate it slowly. Evaporate the percolate under reduced pressure and at a temperature not exceeding 60°C to a soft extract, add 50 g of dry starch and continue the evaporation at the same temperature, until the product is dry. Powder the residue.

Label

BELLADONNA EXTRACT USP		
(50 ml)		
Composition:		**Mfg. Lic. No.-** 4H/2010
Each 50 ml contains,	**BELLADON**	**Batch No.-** BN 0115
Belladonna- 5 g	(Extract)	**Mfg. Date-** Feb. 2011
Alcohol q.s.- 50 ml	(Used as antispasmodic)	**Exp. Date-** Jan. 2012
		M.R.P.- Rs. 20.00
Storage: Store in tight, light-resistant containers at a temperature not exceeding 30°C.	**PROTECT FROM SUN LIGHT**	(Inclusive of all taxes)
		Mfd. By: YAVI PHARMA KANPUR ROAD, LUCKNOW UP- 226001

Marketed Preparations

Active Ingredient(s)	Marketed preparation (Manufacturer)
Benzoin	**BENZOIN TINCTURE** (WALLIS PHARMACEUTICALS), **COMPOUND BENZOIN TINCTURE** (SG LABORATORY), **COMPOUND BENZOIN TINCTURE** (K. PHARMACEUTICAL WORKS), **COMPOUND BENZOIN TINCTURE** (THE SWASTIK PHARMACEUTICALS)
Iodine	**IODINE TINCTURE** (GARIMA HEALTHCARE), **IODINE TINCTURE** (THE SWASTIK PHARMACEUTICALS), **IODINE TINCTURE** (WALLIS PHARMACEUTICALS),
Ashwagandha	**ASHWAGANDHA TINCTURE** (VASUNDHARA BIOTECH)
Cardamom	**COMPOUND CARDAMOM TINCTURE** (THE SWASTIK PHARMACEUTICALS)
Ginger	**GINGER TINCTURE** (K. PHARMACEUTICAL WORKS), **WEAK GINGER TINCTURE** (THE SWASTIK PHARMACEUTICALS), **WEAK GINGER TINCTURE** (DEOGHAR PHARMACEUTICALS)
Orange	**ORANGE TINCTURE** (DEOGHAR PHARMACEUTICALS)

EXERCISE - 20

Object

To prepare and submit 50 ml Infusion of Tea.

Principle

Infusions are usually prepared form vegetable drugs containing water soluble and easily extractable principles. The process consists of moistening the drug with water, macerating it with boiling water and straining and making up the required volume e.g. Concentrated Chirata Infusion and Compound Chirata Infusion, Infusion of Tea. Infusions must be freshly prepared and should be consumed within 24 hours of its preparation.

Formula

Ingredients	Quantity Required
Tea leaves (in coarse powder form)	5 g
Purified water q.s. to	100 ml

Apparatus

Glass beaker, measuring cylinder and volumetric pipette.

Procedure

Weigh the required quantity of tea leaves and place at the bottom of the infusion pot, add water and stir the contents occasionally otherwise the tea leaves may be enclosed in a piece of muslin cloth and suspended just below the level of the water. The drug is allowed to remain in contact with water for about 15 minutes. After the specified time the liquid is strained and dispensed. The marc is not pressed to avoid expression of colloidal cells into the preparation and the final volume of the preparation is not adjusted by adding more of the vehicle otherwise dilution of active constituents will take place.

Category

Stimulant.

Dose

As directed by physician.

Therapeutic Use

Infusion of Tea is used as stimulant of nervous system.

Storage

Infusion of Tea should be stored in well closed container in a cool place.

Label

'SHAKE WELL BEFORE USE'.

Specimen Label

The specimen label for Infusion of Tea is given as:

<table>
<tr><td colspan="3" align="center">INFUSION OF TEA
(50 ml)</td></tr>
<tr>
<td>Composition:
Each 50 ml contains,
Tea leaves (powdered)- 2.5 g
Purified water q.s.- 50 ml
Dose- As directed by physician.
Storage- Store in well closed, amber coloured glass bottle in cool place.</td>
<td align="center">THEA-FUSION
(Infusion)
Stimulant

SHAKE WELL BEFORE USE
NOT FOR INJECTION</td>
<td>Mfg. Lic. No.- 8J/2010
Batch No.- JM 0512
Mfg. Date- May 2011
Exp. Date- Apr. 2012
M.R.P.- Rs. 25.00
(Inclusive of all taxes)
Mfd. By: YAVI PHARMA
KANPUR ROAD,
LUCKNOW UP- 226001</td>
</tr>
</table>

EXERCISE - 21

Object

To prepare and submit 50 ml Decoction of Senna.

Principle

Decoctions are solutions of vegetable principles, obtained by boiling the substances containing these principles in water. All vegetable substances are not suitable for decoction. In many the active principle is volatile at a boiling temperature; in others it undergoes some change unfavorable to its activity. The decoction should always be strained while hot, so that the matter which separates on cooling may be mixed again with the fluid by agitation at the time of administering the remedy.

As a rule, glass or earthenware vessels should be preferred, as those made of metal are sometimes corroded by the ingredients of the decoction, which thus become contaminated. Vessels of block tin are preferable to those made of copper, brass, or zinc; but iron pots should not be used where astringent vegetable substances are concerned.

Decoctions are prone to fermentation hence they should be prepared only when wanted for use, and should not be kept, when the weather is warm, for a longer period than 48 hours.

Senna leaf consists of the dried leaflets of *Cassia senna* (Family- Caesalpiniaceae) known in commerce as Alexandrian senna leaf or *C. angustifolia* (Family- Caesalpiniaceae), known in commerce as Tinnevelly senna leaf or a mixture of both species.

Formula

Ingredients	Quantity Required
Senna leaf (coarsely comminuted)	50 g
Purified water q.s.	1000 ml

Apparatus

Glass beaker, measuring cylinder and volumetric pipette.

Procedure

Decoction must be freshly prepared. Take the required quantity of coarsely comminuted senna leaf and purified water. Place the drug in a suitable vessel provided with a cover, pour upon it 1000 ml of cold water, cover it well, and boil for 15 minutes. Then allow it to cool to about 40°C, express, strain the expressed liquid and pass enough cold water through the strainer to make the product 1000 ml.

Category

Laxative.

Dose

12 to 20 ml.

Therapeutic Use

The Decoction of Senna works as laxative which promote the evacuation of bowels thus used for the treatment of constipation.

Storage

The decoction of senna should be stored in the well closed container and keep in cool and dark place.

Label

'SHAKE WELL BEFORE USE'.

Specimen Label

The specimen label for Decoction of Senna is given as:

<table>
<tr><td colspan="3" align="center">DECOCTION OF SENNA
(50 ml)</td></tr>
<tr>
<td>Composition:
Each 50 ml contains,
Senna leaves (powder)- 2.5 g
Purified water q.s.- 50 ml
Dose: 12 to 20 ml
Storage: Store in well closed, amber colored glass bottle in cool place.</td>
<td align="center">DECOSENNA

(Decoction)

(Used as Laxative)

SHAKE WELL BEFORE USE</td>
<td>Mfg. Lic. No.- 3H/2010
Batch No.- NM 059
Mfg. Date- Mar. 2011
Exp. Date- Feb. 2012
M.R.P.- Rs. 28.00
(Inclusive of all taxes)
Mfd. By: YAVI PHARMA
KANPUR ROAD, LUCKNOW
UP- 226001</td>
</tr>
</table>

EXERCISE - 22

Object

To prepare and submit 50 ml Compound Benzoin Tincture BP.

Principle

Tinctures are alcoholic or hydroalcoholic solutions usually containing relatively low concentration of the active principles of vegetable drugs or animal drugs. When only one drug is used for making a tincture it is simply designated as Tincture but when more than one vegetable or animal drug is used, the preparation is known as Compound Tincture. Tinctures vary widely in their method of preparation, the strength of active ingredients, their alcohol content and their intended use in medicine and pharmaceutical field.

Compound Benzoin Tincture BP is also knows as Friars' Balsam. It is an extemporaneous preparation. The content of total balsamic acids in Compound Benzoin Tincture BP is not less than 4.5% w/v, calculated as cinnamic acid; ethanol content is 70 to 76% v/v and relative density is 0.880 to 0.910.

Formula

Ingredients	Quantity Required
Barbados aloes / Cape aloes	20 g
Prepared storax of commerce	100 g
Sumatra benzoin crushed	100 g
Ethanol (90%) q.s. to	1000 ml

Apparatus

Glass beaker, measuring cylinder and volumetric pipette.

Procedure

Weigh the required quantity of all ingredients. Macerate the Barbados aloes or Cape aloes, the prepared storax and the Sumatra benzoin with 800 ml of ethanol (90%) in a closed vessel for not less than 2 days, shaking occasionally, filter and pass sufficient ethanol (90%) through the filter to produce 1000 ml. Transfer in clean amber colored glass container and close it tightly.

Category

Protective.

Dose

2 to 4 ml.

Therapeutic Use

Compound Benzoin Tincture BP is used to protect and toughen skin in the treatment of bad sores, ulcers, cracked nipples and fissures of the lips and anus. It is used as an antiseptic and styptic dressing for small cuts by applying undiluted upon lint. It is also used with hot water for inhalation in bronchitis and inflammatory conditions of the pharynx and larynx, and is given internally in chronic bronchitis.

Storage

Store in well-closed, light resistant container in cool place to prevent the volatilization of active ingredients.

Label

'PROTECT FROM SUN LIGHT' to protect the volatile constituents in the preparation.

Specimen Label

The specimen label for Compound Benzoin Tincture BP is given as:

<table>
<tr><td colspan="3" align="center">COMPOUND BENZOIN TINCTURE BP
(50 ml)</td></tr>
<tr>
<td>Composition:
Each 50 ml contains,
Barbados Aloes- 1 g
Sumatra Benzoin- 5 g
Prepared storax- 5 g
Ethanol (90%) q.s.- 50 ml
Dose: 2 to 4 ml
Storage: Store in well closed, amber colored glass bottle in cool place.</td>
<td align="center">COM-BENZ TINCTURE
(Tincture)
(Used as Protective)

FOR EXTERNAL USE ONLY
SHAKE WELL BEFORE USE
PROTECT FROM SUN LIGHT</td>
<td>Mfg. Lic. No.- 2D/2010
Batch No.- FG 032
Mfg. Date- Aug. 2011
Exp. Date- July 2012
M.R.P.- Rs. 35.00
(Inclusive of all taxes)
Mfd. By: YAVI PHARMA
KANPUR ROAD, LUCKNOW UP- 226001</td>
</tr>
</table>

EXERCISE - 23

Object

To prepare and submit 50 ml Strong Ginger Tincture BP.

Principle

Ginger consists of rhizome of *Zingiber officinale* (Family- Zingibracae). The oleo-resins present in the ginger are not soluble in water or dilute alcohol hence strong alcohol must be used to effect extraction. It is prepared by percolation process. Ginger (in moderately coarse powder) is used to expose an adequately large surface to the solvent action of the menstruum. Before packing the drug into the percolator, moistening is done to swell drug otherwise if the swelling takes place in the percolator it will lead to tight packing of the drug and percolation would not taker place properly. After packing the moistened drug in the percolator, sufficient menstruum is poured and allowed to set aside for 24 hours so that the soluble matter can pass into the solution. The marc is pressed to recover the menstruum up to maximum extent. Filtration is done to remove the cell debris expelled by expression of the marc.

Strong Ginger Tincture BP contains 80% to 88% v/v ethanol and relative density between 0.832 to 0.846.

Formula

Ingredients	Quantity Required
Ginger (moderately coarse powder)	500 g
Ethanol (90%) q.s. to	1000 ml

Apparatus

Glass beaker, measuring cylinder, percolator.

Procedure

Moisten the ginger with a portion of menstruum and set aside for 4 to 6 hours. Pack the moistened drug in the percolator. Pour sufficient menstruum on to the ginger to saturate the column of drug throughout its length and also form a layer above it. Set aside for 24 hours. Commence the percolation and collect the percolate in the vessel. Continue percolation until ¾th of volume of the finished product is obtained. Press the marc and add the expressed liquid to the already collected percolate. The total volume should be about 80 to 90% of the final volume. Add more of menstruum to produce the required volume. Allow the liquid to stand to settle the suspended particles. Decant or clarify the liquid by filtration.

Category

Carminative and flavoring agent.

Dose

0.3 to 0.6 ml.

Therapeutic Use

It is used as carminative and flavoring agent.

Storage

Store in well-closed, light resistant container in cool place to prevent the volatilization and deterioration (photochemical changes) of active constituents.

Label

'PROTECT FROM SUN LIGHT'.

Specimen Label

The specimen label for Strong Ginger Tincture BP is given as

<table>
<tr><td colspan="3" align="center">STRONG GINGER TINCTURE BP
(50 ml)</td></tr>
<tr>
<td>Composition:
Each 50 ml contains,
Ginger- 25 g
Ethanol (90%) q.s.- 50 ml
Dose: 0.3 to 0.6 ml.
Storage: Store in well closed, amber colored glass bottle in cool place.</td>
<td align="center">YAVIGIN TINCTURE
(Tincture)
(Used as carminative and Flavoring agent)

PROTECT FROM SUN LIGHT
SHAKE WELL BEFORE USE</td>
<td>Mfg. Lic. No.- 2K/2010
Batch No.- HT 0512
Mfg. Date- Aug. 2011
Exp. Date- July 2012
M.R.P.- Rs. 25.00
(Inclusive of all taxes)
Mfd. By: YAVI PHARMA
KANPUR ROAD,
LUCKNOW UP- 226001</td>
</tr>
</table>

EXERCISE - 24

Object

To prepare and submit 50 ml Liquorice Liquid Extract BP.

Principle

Liquorice consists of the dried peeled root and peeled underground stem of *Glycyrrhiza glabra* (Family- Leguminosae).

Liquid extracts are prepared by using ethanol of suitable concentration or water to extract the herbal drug or animal matter, or by dissolving a soft or dry extract (which has been produced using the same strength of extraction solvent as is used in preparing the liquid extract by direct extraction) of the herbal drug or animal matter in either ethanol of suitable concentration or water. Thus Liquorice Liquid Extract BP is prepared by extracting Liquorice with purified water and adding sufficient ethanol (90%) to give an ethanol content of 18% v/v in the final extract. It is an extemporaneous preparation. Its ethanol content is 16% to 20% v/v and relative density is 1.125 to 1.140.

Formula

Ingredients	Quantity Required
Liquorice (unpeeled, in coarse powder)	1000 g
Purified water	q.s.
Ethanol (90%)	q.s.

Apparatus

Glass beaker, measuring cylinder and volumetric pipette.

Procedure

Exhaust the liquorice with purified water by percolation. Boil the percolate for 5 minutes and set aside for not less than 12 hours. Decant the clear liquid, filter the remainder, mix the two liquids and evaporate until the weight per ml of the liquid is 1.198 g. Add to this liquid, when cold, one quarter of its volume of ethanol (90%). Allow to stand for not less than 4 weeks and then filter. Transfer it in clean amber colored glass container and close it tightly.

Category

Mild expectorant.

Dose

2 to 4 ml.

Therapeutic Use

Liquorice Liquid Extract BP is used in cough mixtures and to disguise the taste of nauseous medicines, especially the alkali iodides, ammonium chloride, quinine and liquid extract of cascara. It can be used as a non-sucrose sweetener, and can be taken safely by diabetics. It is also used in bronchial problems such as catarrh, bronchitis and coughs. It reduces irritation of the throat and yet has an expectorant action. It is a potent healing agent for tuberculosis.

It has a marked effect upon the endocrine system. Its glycosides are structurally similar to the natural steroids of the body, and are responsible for the beneficial action that this herb has in the treatment of adrenal gland problems such as Addison's disease.

Storage

Store in well-closed container in cool place.

Label

'SHAKE WELL BEFORE USE'.

Caution

Long-term usage at high doses of Liquorice Liquid Extract BP may cause sodium retention, low potassium levels and hypertension.

Specimen Label

The specimen label for Liquorice Liquid Extract BP is given as:

LIQUORICE LIQUID EXTRACT BP (50 ml)		
Composition: Each 50 ml contains, Liquorice- 5 g Purified water- q.s. Ethanol (90%) q.s.- 50 ml **Dose:** 2 to 4 ml. **Storage:** Store in well closed, amber colored container in cool place.	**LIQUOR** (Liquid Extract) (Used as expectorant) **SHAKE WELL BEFORE USE**	**Mfg. Lic. No.-** 6J/2010 **Batch No.-** BJ 089 **Mfg. Date-** Aug. 2011 **Exp. Date-** Sep. 2012 **M.R.P.-** Rs. 32.00 (Inclusive of all taxes) **Mfd. By:** YAVI PHARMA KANPUR ROAD, LUCKNOW UP- 226001

CHAPTER 13

PASTES

Pastes are semisolid preparations for external use. They consist of finely powdered medicaments combined with white soft paraffin or liquid paraffin or with a non-greasy base made from glycerol, mucilages or soaps. Pastes contain a high proportion of powdered ingredients so they are normally very stiff therefore they do not spread easily which localizes drug delivery. This is particularly important if the ingredient to be applied on the skin is corrosive such as dithranol, coal tar or salicylic acid. It is easier to apply a paste to a discrete skin area such as a particular lesion or plaque and therefore do not compromise the integrity of healthy skin.

Pastes are useful for absorbing harmful chemicals like ammonia which is released by bacterial action on urine and so are often used in nappy products. Due to high powder content, they are often used to absorb wound exudates. Pastes are thick hence form an unbroken and opaque layer over the skin which acts as a sun filter. This property of pastes makes them suitable for use for skiers as they prevent excessive dehydration of the skin (wind burn) in addition to sun blocking.

Advantages

1. Due to the high solids content, pharmaceutical pastes are often porous, allowing moisture loss from the applied site.
2. Pastes may absorb moisture and chemicals within the exudates.
3. The opaque nature of pastes enables this formulation to be used as a sun block.
4. The chemical stability of therapeutic agents that are prone to hydrolysis will be dramatically enhanced by formulation within pharmaceutical ointments and pastes.

Disadvantages

1. Pastes are generally applied as a thick layer at the required site and are therefore considered to be cosmetically unacceptable.

167

2. Staining of clothes is often associated with the use of pharmaceutical pastes.

3. The viscosity of pastes may be problematic in their spreading over the affected site.

4. They are generally not applied to the hair due to difficulties associated with removal.

Topically applied pastes are non-sterile products; however, they are manufactured under hygienic conditions to minimize the microbial bioburden within the formulated product. Pastes do not contain water so the addition of a preservative is usually not required due to the low water activity in the formulation. But if the product contains water, then a preservative will be required. Preservatives that may be used in pastes include- phenolics e.g. phenol (0.2-0.5%) and chlorocresol (0.075-0.12%), benzoic acid and salts (0.1-0.3%), methylparabens (0.02-0.3%), propylparabens (0.02-0.3%), benzyl alcohol (3.0%), phenoxyethanol (0.5-1.0%) and bronopol (0.01-0.1%).

Paste Bases

Three types of bases are usually employed in the formulation of pastes-

(i)   Hydrocarbon bases

These bases include various paraffins like soft paraffin, hard paraffin and liquid paraffin. These bases are used in varying proportions to get a desirable consistency.

(ii) Water miscible bases

These are hydrous, hydrophilic, oil in water (o/w) emulsion bases e.g. Emulsifying ointment is used as a base for Resorcinol and Sulphur Paste BPC and Emulsifying wax is used in the preparation of Zinc and Coal tar Paste.

(iii) Water soluble bases

These bases are prepared by the use of macrogols of different molecular weights. High molecular weight macrogols are solids while low molecular weight macrogols are liquids.

Methods of Preparation

The manufacturing of pastes is similar to that of emulsions and creams. The simplest method involves the dispersal of the powdered therapeutic agents into the preheated hydrocarbon base using a mechanical mixer. Heat is required to lower the viscosity of the base, thereby facilitating the mixing of the solid drug. Pastes can be prepared by two methods:

(A) Fusion method

This method is employed when the base is semisolid. All the ingredients are fused in a beaker on a water bath and stirred well to mix and cool.

(B) Trituration method

This method is used when the vehicle is a liquid or when the base is semisolid.

In both the methods, either tile and spatula or mortar and pestle are used.

Therapeutic Uses

The use of pastes is generally reserved for certain topical conditions, e.g. the treatment of warts. The principal use of pastes is traditionally as an antiseptic, protective or soothing dressing. Often before application the paste was spread on lint and then applied as a dressing.

Dose

Apply to the affected areas once or twice daily or as directed by physician.

Storage Conditions

The pastes should be stored in a well closed container in a cool place. A collapsible tube or plain amber jar would be most suitable.

Specific Labeling Requirement

'FOR EXTERNAL USE ONLY, 'KEEP OUT OF THE REACH OF CHILDREN' and 'PROTECT FROM SUNLIGHT'.

Examples of Some Pastes

1. Compound Zinc Paste BP

It is used to treat nappy and urinary rash and eczematous conditions and also forms an effective sun block.

Composition	Method of Preparation
Zinc oxide- 25 g Starch- 25 g White soft paraffin- 50 g	Weigh the required quantity of zinc oxide, starch and white soft paraffin. Transfer zinc oxide to a porcelain mortar, add starch to the mortar and triturate with the pestle to form an evenly mixed powder. Transfer the powder and white soft paraffin to a glass tile. Mix the powders with the white soft paraffin using a metal spatula by doubling up method. Triturate until a smooth product is formed.

Label

<table>
<tr><td colspan="3" align="center">COMPOUND ZINC PASTE BP
(50 g)</td></tr>
<tr>
<td>Composition:
Each 50 g contains,
Zinc oxide- 12.5 g
Starch- 12.5 g
White soft paraffin q.s- 50 g
Dose: As directed by physician
Storage: Store in a well closed light resistant container in a cool place.</td>
<td align="center">STARZIN
(Paste)
(Used as mild astringent)

PROTECT FROM SUN LIGHT
FOR EXTERNAL USE ONLY</td>
<td>Mfg. Lic. No.- 5G/2010
Batch No.- BH 320
Mfg. Date- June 2011
Exp. Date- May 2012
M.R.P.- Rs. 22.00
(Inclusive of all taxes)
Mfd. By: ROBIN PHARMA MATHURA ROAD, ALIGARH, UP.</td>
</tr>
</table>

2. Compound Aluminium Paste (Baltimore Paste) BPC

It is used to protect the skin and prevent maceration around colostomies and ileostomies.

Composition	Method of Preparation
Aluminium (powder)- 200 g Zinc oxide- 400 g Liquid paraffin q.s.- 1000 g	Sieve the aluminium (powder) and the zinc oxide. Mix the powders using the 'doubling-up' technique. Mix the powders with the liquid paraffin, stirring until a smooth product is formed.

Label

<table>
<tr><td colspan="3" align="center">COMPOUND ALUMINIUM PASTE (BALTIMORE PASTE) BPC
(50 g)</td></tr>
<tr>
<td>Composition:
Each 50 g contains,
Aluminium (powder)- 10 g
Zinc oxide- 20 g
Liquid paraffin q.s.- 50 g
Dose: As directed by physician
Storage: Store in tight, light-resistant container in a cool place.</td>
<td align="center">COMLUMIN
(Paste)
(Used as a protective)

PROTECT FROM SUN LIGHT
FOR EXTERNAL USE ONLY</td>
<td>Mfg. Lic. No.- 4J/2010
Batch No.- MN 122
Mfg. Date- July 2011
Exp. Date- June 2012
M.R.P.- Rs. 20.00
(Inclusive of all taxes)
Mfd. By: RAVI PHARMA VARANASI UP.</td>
</tr>
</table>

3. Zinc and Coal Tar Paste (White's Tar Paste) BP

Composition	Method of Preparation	Alternative Method of Preparation
Zinc oxide (finely sifted)- 60 g Coal tar- 60 g Emulsifying wax- 50 g Starch- 380 g Yellow soft paraffin q.s.- 1000 g	Melt the yellow soft paraffin and emulsifying wax at the lowest possible temperature. Mix well and stir until just setting. Mix the powders using the 'doubling-up' technique. Levigate the semi-molten base with the powders on a warmed tile. Finally, incorporate the coal tar. The emulsifying wax is added to help in the dispersal of coal tar through the product. This method reduces the amount of heat to which the coal tar is exposed because the constituents of coal tar tend to precipitate out quickly on heating.	Melt the yellow soft paraffin and emulsifying wax together at the lowest possible temperature, stir until cool, to make a homogeneous product. Mix the powders into the base on a glass tile using a spatula. Finally, incorporate the coal tar. This method would avoid heating of coal tar and therefore prevents the volatilization of some of the coal tar constituents and reduces the risk of sedimentation.

Label

ZINC AND COALTAR PASTE (WHITE'S TAR PASTE) BP (50 g)		
Composition: Each 50 g contains, Zinc oxide (finely sifted)- 3 g Coal tar- 3 g Emulsifying wax- 2.5 g Starch- 19 g Yellow soft paraffin q.s.- 50 g **Dose:** Once or twice daily **Storage:** Store in tight, light-resistant container in a cool place.	**ZINCOTAR** (Paste) (Used as an antipruritic agent and to treat psoriasis) **PROTECT FROM SUN LIGHT** **FOR EXTERNAL USE ONLY**	**Mfg. Lic. No.-** 2J/2010 **Batch No.-** FL 291 **Mfg. Date-** Nov. 2011 **Exp. Date-** Oct. 2012 **M.R.P.-** Rs. 24.00 (Inclusive of all taxes) **Mfd. By:** DOLPHIN PHARMA JODHPUR, RAJASTHAN

4. Zinc and Salicylic acid Paste (Lassar's Paste) BP

Composition	Method of Preparation
Zinc oxide- 240 g Salicylic acid- 20 g Starch- 240 g White soft paraffin- 500 g	Weigh the required quantity of zinc oxide, salicylic acid, starch and white soft paraffin. Transfer zinc oxide, salicylic acid and starch to a porcelain mortar and triturate to form an evenly mixed powder. Transfer the powder and white soft paraffin to a glass tile and mix using a metal spatula by doubling up method. Triturate until a smooth paste is formed.

Label

ZINC AND SALICYLIC ACID PASTE (LASSAR'S PASTE) BP (50 g)		
Composition: Each 50 g contains, Zinc oxide- 12 g Salicylic acid- 1 g Starch- 12 g White soft paraffin q.s.- 50 g **Dose:** Apply twice a day **Storage:** Store in tight, light-resistant container in a cool place.	**ZINSAL** (Paste) (Used for hyperkeratosis) **PROTECT FROM SUN LIGHT** **FOR EXTERNAL USE ONLY**	**Mfg. Lic. No.-** 4M/2010 **Batch No.-** SA 012 **Mfg. Date-** Sep. 2011 **Exp. Date-** Aug. 2012 **M.R.P.-** Rs. 22.00 (Inclusive of all taxes) **Mfd. By:** PRAVI PHARMA KANPUR ROAD, LUCKNOW UP- 226001

5. Dithranol Paste BP

The strength of dithranol in paste can vary between 0.1% and 1%. Dithranol is extremely irritant and care should be taken when handling. If large quantities are to be made, the use of liquid paraffin to dissolve the powder prior to addition to the paste reduces the possibility of dispersal of the powder when admixing with the paste. If used, the formula would need to be slightly adjusted to allow for the weight of liquid paraffin used. It is used in treatment of subacute and chronic psoriasis.

Composition	Method of Preparation
Dithranol- 0.1 g Zinc and Salicylic acid Paste q.s.- 100 g	Weigh dithranol and zinc and salicylic acid paste. Transfer them to a warm glass tile and triturate by 'doubling up' method until a smooth product is formed.

Label

DITHRANOL PASTE BP (50 g)		
Composition: Each 50 g contains, Dithranol- 0.05 g Zinc and salicylic acid paste q.s.- 50 g **Dose:** As directed by physician. **Storage:** Store in tight, light-resistant container in a cool place.	**DIZISAL** (Paste) (Used in the treatment of psoriasis) **PROTECT FROM SUN LIGHT** **FOR EXTERNAL USE ONLY** **KEEP OUT OF THE REACH OF CHILDREN**	**Mfg. Lic. No.-** 4D/2010 **Batch No.-** BH 321 **Mfg. Date-** July 2011 **Exp. Date-** June 2012 **M.R.P.-** Rs. 28.00 (Inclusive of all taxes) **Mfd. By:** MOZILLA PHARMA KANPUR ROAD, JHANSI, UP- 284301

6. Coal Tar Paste BP

Composition	Method of Preparation
Strong coal tar solution- 75 g Compound zinc paste- 925 g	Triturate the strong coal tar solution with a portion of the compound zinc paste until smooth and gradually incorporate the remainder of the compound zinc paste.

Label

COAL TAR PASTE BP (50 g)		
Composition: Each 50 g contains, Strong coal tar solution- 3.75 g Compound zinc paste q.s.- 50 g **Dose:** As directed by physician. **Storage:** Store in tight, light-resistant container in a cool place.	**COTAR-PASTE** (Paste) (Used in the treatment of psoriasis) **PROTECT FROM SUN LIGHT** **FOR EXTERNAL USE ONLY**	**Mfg. Lic. No.-** 2G/2010 **Batch No.-** NM 297 **Mfg. Date-** Apr. 2011 **Exp. Date-** Mar. 2012 **M.R.P.-** Rs. 22.00 (Inclusive of all taxes) **Mfd. By:** YAVI PHARMA KANPUR ROAD, LUCKNOW UP- 226001

Marketed Preparations

Active Ingredient(s)	Marketed Preparation (Manufacturer)
Zinc and Salicylic acid	**ZINC AND SALICYLIC ACID PASTE (LESSAR'S PASTE)** (AGRAWAL PHARMACEUTICALS), **ZINC AND SALICYLIC ACID PASTE (LESSAR'S PASTE)** (ALPINE INDUSTRIES)
Potassium nitrate	**ACCENT** (ZEE LAB), **SENQUEL** (DR. REDDY'S LAB), **TRIGUARD** (FDC), **LEDENT** (LEXUS)
Strontium chloride	**EXELENT** (ZEE LAB)

EXERCISE - 25

Object

To prepare and submit 50 g of Zinc Gelatin Paste (Unna's Paste) BPC.

Principle

Pastes are semisolid preparations containing a high proportion of finely powdered medicaments and are meant for external application. They are characterized by a definite yield value and increase in the resistance to flow with increased force of application. They are usually stiffer, less greasy and more absorptive as compared to the ointments. As they absorb serum secretions, pastes are used for acute lesions having an oozing tendency. Pastes are mainly used as vehicles for astringent and antiseptic agents.

Formula

Ingredients	Quantity Required
Zinc oxide (finely sifted)	150 g
Gelatin	150 g
Glycerol	350 g
Purified water q.s. to	1000 g

Apparatus

Glass beaker, measuring cylinder and knife.

Procedure

Weigh the required quantities of zinc oxide (finely sifted), gelatin and glycerol. Add the gelatin in boiled purified water and stir gently until dissolved. Add the glycerol (previously heated to a temperature not higher than 100°C) and stir gently to prevent incorporation of air bubbles until solution is complete. Maintain the base at 100°C for 1 hour to remove any microbial contamination. Adjust the base to weight by evaporation or adding hot purified water as required. Sift the zinc oxide and add in small amounts of molten base. Continue stirring until the preparation is viscous enough to support the powder but is still pourable. Pour into a shallow tray, allow to set and cut up into cubes. Cutting of paste into cubes reduces the tendency of the zinc oxide to sediment out.

The preparation is designed to be re-melted before application as a dressing for varicose ulcers. Re-melting is achieved by standing the container in hot water. The gel reforms on cooling.

Category

Astringent.

Dose

As directed by physician.

Therapeutic Use

It is used as an absorbent and mild astringent.

Storage

Unna's Paste should be stored in tight, light-resistant container in a cool place.

Label

'PROTECT FROM SUNLIGHT'.

Specimen Label

The specimen label for Unna's Paste BPC is given as:

<table>
<tr><td colspan="3" align="center">ZINC GELATIN PASTE (UNNA'S PASTE) BPC
(50 g)</td></tr>
<tr>
<td>Composition:
Each 50 g contains,
Zinc oxide- 7.5 g
Gelatin- 7.5 g
Glycerol- 17.5 g
Purified water q.s.- 50 g
Dose: As directed by physician.
Storage: Store in tight, light-resistant container in cool place.</td>
<td align="center">ZINGEL
(Paste)
(Used as an absorbent and mild astringent)

PROTECT FROM SUN LIGHT</td>
<td>Mfg. Lic. No.- 4H/2010
Batch No.- JH 210
Mfg. Date- Sep. 2011
Exp. Date- Aug. 2012
M.R.P.- Rs. 25.00
(Inclusive of all taxes)
Mfd. By: KALPI PHARMA KANPUR ROAD, JHANSI, UP- 284301.</td>
</tr>
</table>

CHAPTER 14

JELLIES

Jellies are transparent or translucent non-greasy semisolid to thick viscous fluids containing submicroscopic particles in a somewhat plastic or rigid vehicle meant for external application to the skin or mucous membrane. These can be prepared by either natural gums e.g. Tragacanth, pectin, alginates or synthetic derivatives of natural substances (e.g. Methylcellulose, sodium carboxymethylcellulose).

Jellies are easy to apply and the evaporation of water content produces a cooling sensation at the site of application. After evaporation of water content jellies stick well to the applied area and provide protection. These can easily be removed by washing with water.

Types of jellies

There are three types of jellies

1. Medicated Jellies

These are mainly used on skin and mucous membrane for their spermicidal, anaesthetic and antiseptic properties e.g. Ephedrine sulphate jelly is used as a vasoconstrictor to stop the bleeding from nose. Phenyl mercuric nitrate jelly is used as a spermicidal contraceptive. Spermicidal agents commonly incorporated in contraceptive jellies are phenylmercuric acetate, nonylphenoxypolyethoxyethanol and paraformaldehyde.

2. Lubricating Jellies

These jellies are used for lubricating the diagnostic equipments, surgical gloves, catheters, rectal thermometers etc. These jellies should be sterile because these are used as lubricant for instruments that are inserted into the various organs of the body like urinary bladder.

3. Miscellaneous Jellies

(a) Patch testing

These jellies are used as a vehicle for allergens, which are applied on the skin to check the sensitivity.

(b) Electrocardiography

The jelly is used on the electrode to reduce the electrical resistance between the patient's skin and the electrode.

Since jellies contain carbohydrates and water as base therefore these are prone to microbial growth so jellies must be suitably preserved.

Methods of Preparation

Pharmaceutical jellies are usually prepared by adding a thickening agent to an aqueous solution of drug. The mass is triturated in a mortar until a uniform product is formed. For the preparation of jellies a whole gum is preferred rather than the powdered gum because the former gives a clear preparation of uniform consistency. The following jelling agents are used for the preparation of jellies-

(a) Tragacanth

It is used for the preparation of lubricating, medicated and contraceptive jellies. The amount of gum required for the preparation of the jelly depends on the intended use of the jelly e.g. for the lubricating jellies 2-3% w/v but for medicated jellies about 5% w/v gum is required. Tragacanth jellies vary in viscosity.

(b) Sodium alginate

Sodium alginate jellies are used as lubricant and dermatological vehicles. For lubricants 1.5-2% w/v and for dermatological vehicles 5-10% w/v sodium alginate is used. It has an advantage over tragacanth as it is available in several grades of standardized viscosity.

(c) Pectin

It is an excellent gelling agent and is used in the preparation of various jellies including edible jellies.

(d) Gelatin

It is soluble in hot water. A hot solution containing only 2% w/v gelatin forms a jelly on cooling. Very stiff medicated jellies can be prepared by incorporating about 15% w/v gelatin. Such jellies are melted before use and after cooling to a desired temperature are used with a brush to the affected area.

(e) Cellulose derivatives

Methylcellulose and sodium carboxymethylcellulose are widely used for the preparation of neutral jellies of very stable viscosity. These jellies are quite clear and after drying form a strong film on the skin. Sodium carboxymethylcellulose is used for the preparation of lubricating jellies as well as sterile jellies.

Since all the jellies contain a large amount of water therefore these must be suitably preserved by adding a suitable preservative e.g. Methyl p-hydroxybenzoate (0.1-0.2% w/v) is commonly used as preservative for medicated jellies.

Therapeutic Uses

These are chiefly used on mucous membrane for their lubricating, antiseptic or spermicidal purposes and also in haemorrhoids.

Dose

As directed by physician.

Storage Conditions

Jellies should be stored in well closed containers in a cool place to minimize the evaporation of water.

Specific Labeling Requirement

'FOR EXTERNAL USE ONLY' and 'PROTECT FROM SUNLIGHT'.

Examples of Some Jellies

1. Ichthammol Jelly

Composition	Method of Preparation
Ichthammol- 1 g Tragacanth (powder)- 2.5 g Alcohol (90%)- 5 ml Glycerin- 1 g Purified water q.s.- 50 g	Weigh the required quantity of ingredients. Take alcohol in 100 ml wide mouth jar and add tragacanth. Shake well to mix and add purified water in it as quickly as possible and shake immediately. Separately mix ichthammol, glycerin and some purified water. Add this solution to the mucilage and shake well. Adjust the final weight by adding sufficient purified water, if required and shake well.

Label

<table>
<tr><td colspan="3" align="center">ICHTHAMMOL JELLY
(50 g)</td></tr>
<tr>
<td>Composition:
Each 50 g contains,
Ichthammol- 1 g
Jelly base q.s.- 50 g
Dose: As directed by physician.
Storage: Store in a well closed light-resistant container in a cool place.</td>
<td align="center">ICHMOL
(Jelly)
(Used as mild astringent)

PROTECT FROM SUN LIGHT
FOR EXTERNAL USE ONLY</td>
<td>Mfg. Lic. No.-2/2010
Batch No.- GH 450
Mfg. Date- June 2011
Exp. Date- May 2012
M.R.P.- Rs. 20.00
(Inclusive of all taxes)
Mfd. By: YAVI PHARMA
KANPUR ROAD, LUCKNOW
UP- 226001</td>
</tr>
</table>

2. Zinc Gelatin Jelly

Composition	Method of Preparation
Zinc oxide- 15 g Gelatin- 15 g Glycerin- 35 g Purified water q.s.- 100 g	Weigh the required quantities of zinc oxide (finely sifted), gelatin and glycerin. Soak the gelatin in purified water until thoroughly softened, add the glycerin and heat over water bath until the gelatin is dissolved, adjust the weight to 85 g, if necessary, adding more purified water. Weigh the required quantity of zinc oxide and pass through sieve no. 120 and add it in small amounts of melted base with gentle stirring to avoid excessive incorporation of air. Continue stirring until a uniform viscous product is obtained.

Label

<table>
<tr><td colspan="3" align="center">ZINC GELATIN JELLY
(50 g)</td></tr>
<tr>
<td>Composition:
Each 50 g contains,
Zinc oxide- 7.5 g
Jelly base q.s.- 50 g
Dose: As directed by physician.
Storage: Store in tight, light-resistant container in a cool place.</td>
<td align="center">ZINGEL
(Jelly)
(Used as a mild astringent)

PROTECT FROM SUN LIGHT
FOR EXTERNAL USE ONLY</td>
<td>Mfg. Lic. No.- 2D/2010
Batch No.- VN 156
Mfg. Date- Aug. 2011
Exp. Date- July 2012
M.R.P.- Rs. 28.00
(Inclusive of all taxes)
Mfd. By: YAVI PHARMA
KANPUR ROAD, LUCKNOW
UP- 226001</td>
</tr>
</table>

3. Methylcellulose Jelly

Composition	Method of Preparation
Methylcellulose (4000 cps)- 0.8 g Carbopol 934- 0.24 g Propylene glycol- 16 g Methyl paraben- 0.015 g Sodium hydroxide solution (pH-7) q.s.- 100 g	Disperse the methylcellulose in hot water, cool it and disperse the carbopol in purified water. Adjust the pH 7 by adding sufficient 1% w/v solution of sodium hydroxide. Dissolve methyl paraben in propylene glycol. Mix the methylcellulose, carbopol and propylene glycol fractions, taking caution to avoid the incorporation of air.

Label

METHYLCELLULOSE JELLY		
(50 g)		
Composition: Each 50 g contains, Methylcellulose- 0.4 g Carbopol 934- 0.12 g Propylene glycol- 8 g Methyl paraben- 0.08 g Sodium hydroxide solution q.s.- 50 g **Storage:** Store in tight, light-resistant container in a cool place.	**METHYLGEL** (Jelly) (Used as lubricating jelly) **PROTECT FROM SUN LIGHT** **FOR EXTERNAL USE ONLY**	**Mfg. Lic. No.-6T/2010** **Batch No.-** FN 182 **Mfg. Date-** Sep. 2011 **Exp. Date-** Aug. 2012 **M.R.P.-** Rs. 18.00 (Inclusive of all taxes) **Mfd. By:** YAVI PHARMA KANPUR ROAD, LUCKNOW UP- 226001

Marketed Preparations

Active Ingredient(s)	Marketed Preparation (Manufacturer)
Gentian violet	**GENTIAN VIOLET JELLY** (ARORA PHARMACEUTICAL PVT LTD)
Clotrimazole	**CANDID- V GEL** (GLENMARK), **CLOMAX VAGINAL GEL** (BOMBAY TABLET)
Lincomycin	**ZYNX GEL** (WALLACE)
Xylocaine	**XYLOCAINE** (ASTRA ZENECA)
Miconazole	**GYNO-DAKTARIN** (ETHNOR PHARMA)

EXERCISE - 26

Object

To prepare and submit 50 g of Sodium Alginate Jelly.

Principle

Pharmaceutical jellies are transparent or translucent semisolid to thick viscous fluids containing submicroscopic particles and used for external application to the skin or mucous membrane. Jellies are generally prepared by triturating a thickening agent to an aqueous solution of drug until a uniform product is formed. Since jellies contain a large amount of water, these are prone to the microbial growth hence must be suitably preserved by adding a suitable preservative e.g. Methyl p-hydroxybenzoate (0.1-0.2% w/v) is commonly used as preservative for medicated jellies.

Formula

Ingredients	Quantity Required
Sodium alginate	7 g
Glycerin	7 g
Methyl hydroxybenzoate	0.2 g
Calcium gluconate	0.05 g
Purified water (freshly boiled and cooled) q.s. to	100 g

Apparatus

Glass beaker, measuring cylinder, glass mortar and pastle.

Procedure

Wet sodium alginate with glycerin in a glass mortar. Dissolve methyl hydroxybenzoate and calcium gluconate in about $^3/_4{}^{th}$ of the purified water (freshly boiled and cooled) with the aid of heat. Cool to about 60°C and stir well. Add sodium alginate and glycerin mixture to it in small proportions, stir vigorously to get uniform product.

Category

Lubricating jelly.

Dose

As directed by physician.

Therapeutic Use

It is used to assist in medical procedures.

Storage

Sodium alginate jelly should be stored in tight, light-resistant container in a cool place.

Label

'PROTECT FROM SUNLIGHT', 'FOR EXTERNAL USE ONLY'.

Specimen Label

The specimen label for Sodium Alginate Jelly is given as:

<table>
<tr><td colspan="3" align="center">SODIUM ALGINATE JELLY
(50 g)</td></tr>
<tr>
<td>Composition:
Each 50 g contains,
Sodium alginate- 3.5 g
Glycerin- 3.5 g
Methyl hydroxybenzoate- 0.1 g
Calcium gluconate- 0.025 g
Purified water q.s.- 50 g
Dose: As directed by physician.
Storage: Store in tight, light-resistant container in cool place.</td>
<td align="center">SOALGIN
(Jelly)
(Used as lubricating jelly)

PROTECT FROM SUN LIGHT
FOR EXTERNAL USE ONLY</td>
<td>Mfg. Lic. No.- 4H/2010
Batch No.- JH 210
Mfg. Date- Sep. 2011
Exp. Date- Aug. 2012

M.R.P.- Rs. 25.00
(Inclusive of all taxes)
Mfd. By: DOLLY PHARMA, M.G. ROAD SURAT, GUJRAT</td>
</tr>
</table>

CHAPTER 15

EAR PREPARATIONS

Ear preparations are also known as otic or aural products. These are liquid, semisolid or solid preparations intended for instillation, for spraying, for insufflation, for application to the auditory meatus or as an ear wash. Ear preparations usually contain one or more active substances in a suitable vehicle. They may contain excipients, for example, to adjust tonicity or viscosity, to adjust the pH, to increase the solubility of the active substances, to stabilize the preparation or to provide adequate antimicrobial properties. The excipients do not adversely affect the intended medicinal action of the preparation or, at the concentrations used, cause toxicity or undue local irritation. The ear preparations for application to the injured ear, particularly where the eardrum is perforated, or prior to surgery must be sterile, free from antimicrobial preservatives and supplied in single-dose containers.

Ear preparations are supplied in multi-dose or single-dose containers. A suitable administration device may be used to avoid the introduction of contaminants. Aqueous ear preparations supplied in multi-dose containers contain a suitable antimicrobial preservative at a suitable concentration, except where the preparation itself has adequate antimicrobial properties. Sterile ear preparations ensure sterility and avoid the introduction of contaminants and the growth of microorganisms. In the manufacture of ear preparations containing dispersed particles, measures are taken to ensure a suitable and controlled particle size with regard to the intended use.

Ear drops are aqueous or oily solutions or suspensions of one or more medicaments intended for instillation into the outer ear. They may contain suitable auxiliary substances such as buffers, stabilizing agents, dispersing agents, solubilizing agents and agents to adjust the tonicity or viscosity of the preparation. However, if buffering agents are used in preparations intended for use in surgical procedures, care should be taken to ensure that the nature and concentration of the selected agents are suitable. Where the active ingredients are susceptible to oxidative degradation, a suitable antioxidant may be added but care should be taken to ensure compatibility between the antioxidant and the other ingredients of the preparations. Any additive in the preparation should not adversely affect the intended medicinal action nor, at the concentrations used, cause undue local irritation.

Certain ear drops may be supplied in dry, sterile form to be constituted in an appropriate sterile liquid immediately before use. Aqueous preparations supplied in multiple application containers contain suitable antimicrobial preservatives at appropriate concentrations except when the product itself has adequate antimicrobial properties. The antimicrobial preservatives should be compatible with the other ingredients of the preparation and should be effective throughout the period of use of the ear drops. Containers for multiple application preparations should permit the withdrawal of successive doses of the preparation. Such containers should normally hold not more than 10 ml. Ear drops intended for use in surgical procedures or for application to injured ear, are sterile. Such preparations should not contain antimicrobial preservatives and should be packed in single dose containers.

Test for Ear Drops

(a) Particle size

This test is applicable only to ear drops that are suspensions. Briefly, introduce a suitable volume of the ear drops into a counting cell or onto a microscope slide, as appropriate. Scan under a microscope an area corresponding to 10 μg of the solid phase. Scan at least 50 representative fields. Not more than 20 particles have a maximum dimension greater than 25 μm, not more than 10 particles have a maximum dimension greater than 50 μm and none has a maximum dimension greater than 100 μm.

(b) Sterility test

When the label indicates that the ear drops are sterile, it complies with the test for sterility. Droppers supplied separately also comply with these tests. Remove the dropper out of the package using aseptic precautions and transfer it to a tube containing suitable culture medium so that it is completely immersed. Incubate and carry out the tests for sterility on the medium.

Method of Preparation

Ear drops that are solutions are practically clear and free from particles when examined under suitable conditions of visibility. Since ear drops can be a simple solution, suspension or an emulsion hence they can be prepared by their respective methods.

Sterile ear drops are prepared using methods designed to ensure their sterility and to avoid the introduction of contaminants and growth of microorganisms. Ear drops can be sterilized by various methods of sterilization.

Ear drops that are suspensions may show a sediment that readily disperses when shaken. The suspension remains sufficiently dispersed to enable the correct dose to be removed from the container.

Therapeutic Uses

The use of ear drops depends on the incorporated active ingredients. Generally ear drops are applied to soften the ear wax and to treat various bacterial and fungal infections.

Dose

As directed by physician.

Storage Conditions

Ear drops should be packed in well-closed containers. If the preparation is sterile, store in sterile, tightly-closed, tamper-evident containers. Containers should be made from materials that do not cause deterioration of the preparation as a result of diffusion into or across the material of the container or by yielding foreign substances to the preparation.

The container and package of a single application preparation should be such as to maintain sterility of the contents and the applicator up to the time of use. Containers for multiple application preparations should be fitted with an integral dropper or with a screw cap made of suitable material incorporating a dropper and plastic or rubber teat. Alternatively, such a cap assembly may be packed separately.

Specific Labeling Requirement

The label of ear drops should state (1) the names and concentrations in percentages, or weight or volume per ml of the active ingredient(s), (2) the names and concentrations of any added antioxidant, stabilizing agent or antimicrobial preservative, (3) for multiple application containers, the contents should not be used for more than 1 month after opening the container, (4) for multiple application containers, care should be taken to avoid contamination of the contents during use, (5) that the preparation is 'NOT FOR INJECTION', where applicable, (6) the preparation is sterile, and (7) the storage conditions.

Examples of Some Ear Preparations

1. Sodium Bicarbonate Ear Drops BP

Composition	Method of Preparation
Sodium bicarbonate- 5 g Glycerol- 30 ml Purified water q.s.- 100 ml	Dissolve the sodium bicarbonate in about 60 ml of purified water, add glycerol and mix then makeup the volume to 100 ml with purified water and mix.

Label

SODIUM BICARBONATE EAR DROPS BP (10 ml)		
Composition: Each 10 ml contains, Sodium bicarbonate- 0.5 g Glycerol- 3 ml Purified water q.s.- 10 ml **Dose:** As directed by physician. **Storage:** Store in a well-closed light-resistant container, in a cool place.	**SODABICARB** (Ear drops) (Used for softening and removal of ear wax) **NOT FOR INJECTION** **FOR EXTERNAL USE ONLY**	**Mfg. Lic. No.-** 4M/2010 **Batch No.-** FH 412 **Mfg. Date-** June 2011 **Exp. Date-** May 2012 **M.R.P.-** Rs. 18.00 (Inclusive of all taxes) **Mfd. By:** YAVI PHARMA KANPUR ROAD, LUCKNOW UP- 226001

2. Aluminium Acetate Ear Drops IP

It is a clear liquid, contains not less than 1.7% w/v and not more than 1.9% w/v of aluminium and weight per ml is 1.06 to 1.08 g.

Composition	Method of Preparation
Aluminium sulphate- 225 g Calcium carbonate- 100 g Tartaric acid- 45 g Acetic acid (33%)- 250 ml Purified water q.s.- 1000 ml	Dissolve the aluminium sulphate in 600 ml of the purified water, add the acetic acid and then the calcium carbonate mixed with the remainder of the purified water and allow to stand for not less than 24 hours in a cool place, stirring occasionally. Filter, add the tartaric acid to the filtrate and mix.

Label

ALUMINIUM ACETATE EAR DROPS IP (10 ml)		
Composition: Each 10 ml contains, Aluminium sulphate- 2.25 g Calcium carbonate- 1 g Tartaric acid- 0.45 g Acetic acid (33%)- 2.5 ml Purified water q.s.- 10 ml **Dose:** As directed by physician. **Storage:** Store in well-closed container, in a cool place.	**ALUMINTA** (Ear drops) **PROTECT FROM SUN LIGHT** **FOR EXTERNAL USE ONLY** **NOT FOR INJECTION**	**Mfg. Lic. No.-** 2D/2010 **Batch No.-** VN 156 **Mfg. Date-** Aug. 2011 **Exp. Date-** July 2012 **M.R.P.-** Rs. 15.00 (Inclusive of all taxes) **Mfd. By:** LAVA PHARMA JHANSI ROAD, BHOPAL, M.P.

3. Boric acid Ear Drops

Composition	Method of Preparation
Boric acid- 0.1 g Denatured spirit- 3 ml Purified water q.s.- 15 ml	Dissolve the required quantity of boric acid in denatured spirit and add sufficient purified water to make volume to 15 ml. Filter to remove impurities, if any.

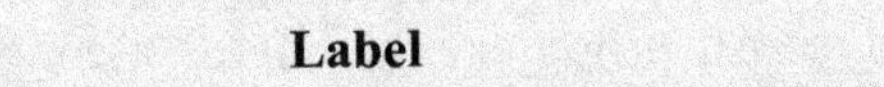

Label

<table>
<tr><td colspan="3" align="center">BORIC ACID EAR DROPS
(15 ml)</td></tr>
<tr>
<td>Composition:
Each 15 ml contains,
Boric acid- 0.1 g
Denatured spirit- 3 ml
Purified water q.s.- 15 ml
Storage: Store in well-closed, light-resistant container, in a cool place.</td>
<td align="center">BOROCID
(Ear drops)
(Used for bacterial infections)

PROTECT FROM SUN LIGHT
FOR EXTERNAL USE ONLY
NOT FOR INJECTION</td>
<td>Mfg. Lic. No.5U/2010
Batch No.- GH 243
Mfg. Date- Nov. 2011
Exp. Date- Oct. 2012
M.R.P.- Rs. 15.00
(Inclusive of all taxes)
Mfd. By: YAVI PHARMA KANPUR ROAD, LUCKNOW UP- 226001</td>
</tr>
</table>

Marketed Preparations:

Active Ingredient(s)	Marketed Preparation (Manufacturer)
Chloramphenicol	**CHLOROMYCETIN** (PFIZER), **BEXY-C** (CADEX LAB), **ENTEROMYCETIN OTIC** (DEY'S), **PARAXIN EAR DROPS** (NICHOLAS PIRAMAL), **XACT** (ZEE LAB)
Gentamicin	**GENTICYN** (NICHOLAS), **BACTIGEN** (FDC)
Beclomethasone	**ADVIN-NC** (ANKARE), **BENTOR** (INDOCO)
Benzocaine	**ANTIWAX** (ZEE LAB)
Ofloxacin	**BESTOFLOX-CL** (BESTOCHEM)

EXERCISE - 27

Object

To prepare and submit 15 ml of Chloramphenicol Ear Drops BP.

Principle

Ear drops are solutions, emulsions or suspensions of one or more active substances in liquids either water, glycerol, propylene glycol or alcohol/water mixtures suitable for application to the auditory meatus without exerting harmful pressure on the ear drum. They may also be placed in the auditory meatus by means of a tampon impregnated with the liquid. Ear drops include antibiotics, antiseptics, cleansing solutions and wax softeners.

Chloramphenicol is sparingly soluble in water but freely soluble in propylene glycol (1 in 7), hence it is used as a vehicle.

Ear drops are usually supplied in multi-dose containers of glass or suitable plastic material that are fitted with an integral dropper or with a screw cap of suitable material incorporating a dropper and rubber or plastic teat. Alternatively, such a cap assembly is supplied separately.

Formula

Ingredients	Quantity Required
Chloramphenicol	0.075 g
Propylene glycol q.s. to	15 ml

Apparatus

Glass beaker and measuring cylinder.

Procedure

It is prepared by simple solution method. Dissolve the required quantity of chloramphenicol in propylene glycol, shake and add remaining quantity of propylene glycol to produce sufficient volume of 15 ml.

Category

Antibiotic.

Dose

Instill 3 drops into the affected ear, 2 times a day or as directed by physician.

Therapeutic Use

It is used in the treatment of chronic otorrhoea and chronic otitis.

Storage

Chloramphenicol Ear Drops BP should be stored in well closed, light-resistant container in a cool place.

Label

'PROTECT FROM SUNLIGHT', 'NOT FOR INJECTION' and 'FOR EXTERNAL USE ONLY'.

Specimen Label

The specimen label for Chloramphenicol Ear Drops BP is given as:

<table>
<tr><td colspan="3">CHLORAMPHENICOL EAR DROPS BP
(15 ml)</td></tr>
<tr>
<td>Composition:
Each 15 ml contains,
Chloramphenicol- 0.075 g
Propylene glycol q.s.- 15 ml
Dose: As directed by physician.
Storage: Store in well-closed, light-resistant container, in cool place.</td>
<td>CHLORAM
(Ear drops)

PROTECT FROM SUN LIGHT
NOT FOR INJECTION
FOR EXTERNAL USE ONLY</td>
<td>Mfg. Lic. No.- 5D/2010
Batch No.- NM 145
Mfg. Date- Sep. 2011
Exp. Date- Aug. 2012
M.R.P.- Rs. 15.00
(Inclusive of all taxes)
Mfd. By: RAJ PHARMA
JHANSI ROAD, LUCKNOW
UP- 226001</td>
</tr>
</table>

CHAPTER 16

EYE PREPARATIONS

Eye preparations are sterile liquid, semisolid or solid preparations intended for administration upon the eyeball and/or to the conjunctiva or for insertion in the conjunctival sac for a local effect. Several categories of eye preparations may be distinguished like eye drops, eye lotions, powders for eye drops and eye lotions, semisolid eye preparations and ophthalmic inserts. Eye-drops are sterile aqueous or oily solutions or suspensions of one or more active substances intended for instillation into the eye.

Eye drops (ophthalmic drops) are sterile, aqueous or oily solutions or suspensions of one or more medicaments intended for instillation into the *cul-de-sac*. They may contain suitable auxiliary substances such as buffers, stabilizing agents, solubilizing agents and agents to adjust the tonicity or viscosity of the preparation. Where the active ingredient is susceptible to oxidative degradation, a suitable antioxidant may be added but care should be taken to ensure compatibility between the antioxidant and the other ingredients of the preparation. Any additive in the preparation should not adversely affect the intended medicinal action nor, at the concentrations used, cause undue local irritation.

Certain eye drops may be supplied in dry, sterile form to be constituted in an appropriate sterile liquid immediately before use. Aqueous preparations supplied in multiple application containers contain suitable antimicrobial preservatives at appropriate concentrations except when the product itself has adequate antimicrobial properties. The antimicrobial preservatives should be compatible with the other ingredients of the preparation and should be effective throughout the period of use of the eye drops. If the preparation does not contain an antimicrobial preservative it should be packed in single application containers. Eye drops intended for use in eye surgery should not contain antimicrobial preservatives and should be packed in single application containers.

Most of the eye drops contain benzalkonium chloride (0.01%), phenyl mercuric nitrate or acetate (0.002%) and chlorhexidine acetate (0.01%) as preservative.

190

Method of Preparation

Eye drops are prepared using methods designed to ensure their sterility and to avoid the introduction of contaminants and growth of microorganisms. In the manufacture of eye preparations containing dispersed particles, measures are taken to ensure a suitable and controlled particle size with regard to the intended use. During the development of an eye preparation, the formulation which contains an antimicrobial preservative, the effectiveness of the chosen preservative shall be demonstrated properly. The preparation of eye drops involves the following general steps-

(a) Dissolution of drug and other additives in a suitable vehicle.

(b) Clarification (filtration) by a suitable method.

(c) Sterilization by a suitable method.

(d) Packing and labeling.

Therapeutic Uses

The use of eye drops depends on the incorporated active ingredients. Eye drops may contain antimicrobial substances like antibiotics, anti-inflammatory agents like corticosteroids, miotic drugs like physostigmine sulphate or mydriatic drug like atropine sulphate.

Dose

Dose is prescribed on the basis of incorporated drug or as directed by physician.

Storage Conditions

Unless otherwise prescribed, store in an airtight, tamper proof sterile container to protect from micro-organisms. Containers should be made from materials that do not cause deterioration of the preparation as a result of diffusion into or across the material of the container or by yielding foreign substances to the preparation. The container and package of a single dose preparation should be such as to maintain sterility of the contents and the applicator up to the time of use.

Containers for multiple application preparations should be fitted with an integral dropper or with a sterile screw cap of suitable materials incorporating a dropper and plastic or rubber teat. Alternatively, such a cap assembly may be packed separately after it is sterilized. Containers of multiple application preparations should permit the withdrawal of successive doses of the preparation. Such containers should normally hold not more than 10 ml.

Specific Labeling Requirement

The label of eye drops should state (1) the names and concentrations in percentages, or weight or volume per ml of the active ingredients, (2) the names and concentrations of any added antimicrobial preservative, (3) the contents should not be used for more than 1 month after opening the container, (4) that the preparation is 'NOT FOR INJECTION', (5) the conditions under which the preparation should be stored, and (6) If any visible particle is seen then discard the preparation.

Examples of Some Eye Preparations

1. Zinc Sulphate Eye Drops BP

Composition	Method of Preparation
Zinc sulphate- 0.025 g Sodium chloride- 0.080 g Purified water q.s.- 10 ml	Dissolve the required quantity of zinc sulphate and sodium chloride in purified water, makeup the volume to10 ml with purified water and mix. Then sterilize the product by autoclaving.

Label

<table>
<tr><td colspan="3" align="center">ZINC SULPHATE EYE DROPS BP
(10 ml)</td></tr>
<tr>
<td>Composition:
Each 10 ml contains,
Zinc sulphate- 0.025 g
Sodium chloride- 0.080 g
Purified water q.s.- 10 ml
Dose: As directed by physician.
Storage: Store in a well-closed container, in a cool place.</td>
<td align="center">SULZIN
(Eye Drops)
(Used as astringent)

NOT FOR INJECTION
FOR EXTERNAL USE ONLY
(The contents should not be used for more than 1 month after the opening of container)</td>
<td>Mfg. Lic. No.- 2H/2010
Batch No.- KA 212
Mfg. Date- July 2011
Exp. Date- June 2012
M.R.P.- Rs. 18.00
(Inclusive of all taxes)
Mfd. By: YANA PHARMA NEW COLONY, UDAIPUR, RAJASTHAN- 313001</td>
</tr>
</table>

2. Atropine Sulphate Eye Drops BP

It is used in iritis, uveitis, cycloplegic refraction procedures, organophosphate poisoning, premedication, and as antispasmodic. The half life of this drop in the eye is long and effects may last for 7 to 12 days after topical application to the eye.

Composition	Method of Preparation
Atropine Sulphate- 0.1 g Sodium chloride- 0.075 g Purified water q.s.- 10 ml	Dissolve the sodium chloride in purified water, add atropine sulphate and dissolve it by shaking. Makeup the volume to 10 ml with purified water and sterilize the product by autoclaving.

Label

<table>
<tr><td colspan="3" align="center">ATROPINE SULPHATE EYE DROPS BP
(10 ml)</td></tr>
<tr>
<td>Composition:
Each 10 ml contains,
Atropine sulphate- 0.1 g
Sodium chloride- 0.075 g
Purified water q.s.- 10 ml
Dose: As directed by physician.
Storage: Store in well-closed container, in a cool place.</td>
<td align="center">ATROSUL
(Eye Drops)
(Used in acute inflammation)

PROTECT FROM SUN LIGHT
FOR EXTERNAL USE ONLY
NOT FOR INJECTION
(The contents should not be used for more than 1 month after the opening of container)</td>
<td>Mfg. Lic. No.- 4F/2010
Batch No.- CH 184
Mfg. Date- Aug. 2011
Exp. Date- July 2012
M.R.P.- Rs. 18.00
(Inclusive of all taxes)
Mfd. By: NITIN PHARMA INDORE ROAD, DEWAS, M.P.</td>
</tr>
</table>

3. Fluorescein Eye Drops BP

Fluorescein sodium is used in ocular diagnostic procedures and for locating damaged areas of the cornea due to injury or disease.

Composition	Method of Preparation
Fluorescein sodium- 0.4 g Sodium chloride- 0.032 g Purified water q.s.- 10 ml	Dissolve the sodium chloride in purified water, add fluorescein sodium and dissolve it by shaking. Makeup the volume to 10 ml with Purified water and sterilize the product by autoclaving.

Label

FLUORESCEIN EYE DROPS BP		
(10 ml)		
Composition:	**FLUORES**	**Mfg. Lic. No.-** 1K/2010
Each 10 ml contains,	(Eye Drops)	**Batch No.-** CN 512
Fluorescein sodium- 0.4 g	(Used as diagnostic aid)	**Mfg. Date-** Sep. 2011
Sodium chloride- 0.032 g		**Exp. Date-** Aug. 2012
Purified water q.s.- 10 ml	**PROTECT FROM SUN LIGHT**	**M.R.P.-** Rs. 20.00
Dose: As directed by physician.	**FOR EXTERNAL USE ONLY**	(Inclusive of all taxes)
Storage: Store in well-closed container, in a cool place.	**NOT FOR INJECTION** *(The contents should not be used for more than 1 month after the opening of container)*	**Mfd. By:** VIDHI PHARMA MEERUT ROAD, KARNAL, HARYANA- 132001

4. Sodium chloride Eye Drops BP

Composition	Method of Preparation
Sodium chloride- 0.09 g Purified water q.s.- 10 ml	Dissolve the sodium chloride in purified water. Clarify by filtration. Makeup the volume to10 ml with purified water and sterilize the product by autoclaving.

Label

SODIUM CHLORIDE EYE DROPS BP		
(10 ml)		
Composition:	*SODICHLOR*	**Mfg. Lic. No.-** 3G/2010
Each 10 mL contains,	(Eye Drops)	**Batch No.-** BH 104
Sodium chloride- 0.09 g	(Used as pharmaceutical aid)	**Mfg. Date-** Oct. 2011
Purified water q.s.- 10 ml		**Exp. Date-** Sep. 2012
Dose: As directed by physician.	**FOR EXTERNAL USE ONLY**	**M.R.P.-** Rs. 10.00
	NOT FOR INJECTION	(Inclusive of all taxes)
Storage: Store in well-closed container, in a cool place.	*(The contents should not be used for more than 1 month after the opening of container)*	**Mfd. By:** JACKSON PHARMA KANPUR ROAD, JHANSI, UP- 284301

Marketed Preparations

Active Ingredient(s)	Marketed preparation (Manufacturer)
Sulphacetamide sodium	**ALBUCID** (ALLERGAN), **ANDREMIDE** (INTAS), **OPTACID** (DEY'S), **ZINCOREN** (INDOCO)
Norfloxacin	**ALFLOX** (ALKEM), **NORWIN** (BESTOCHEM), **NORZY** (ZEE LAB), **NORBACTIN EYE DROPS** (RANBAXY)
Ofloxacin	**ENTOF** (DEY'S), **EXOCIN** (ALLERGAN), **OFLACIN** (MICROVISION), **ZO** (FDC), **OFLOX** (CIPLA)
Ciprofloxacin	**ADIFLOX** (INTAS), **ALCIPRO** (ALKEM), **CIPLOX-D** (CIPLA), **CIPROBID EYE DROPS** (CADILA)
Gentamicin	**CINZY** (ZEE LAB), **TAMIGEN** (INDOCO), **GARAMYCIN** (FULFORD), **GENTICYN** (ALLERGEN)

Note: Some of the marketed products are available as Ear/Eye preparations and hence can be used in ear as well as eye.

EXERCISE - 28

Object

To prepare and submit 10 ml of Pilocarpine Eye Drops BP.

Principle

Eye drops (ophthalmic drops) are sterile, aqueous or oily solutions or suspensions of one or more medicaments intended for instillation into the *cul-de-sac*. They may contain suitable excipients like buffers, stabilizing agents, solubilizing agents, tonicity adjuster and viscosity modifier. Any additive in the preparation should not adversely affect the intended medicinal action nor, at the concentrations used, cause undue local irritation. Pilocarpine nitrate is a white or almost white, crystalline powder or colorless crystals, sensitive to light. It is freely soluble in water but sparingly soluble in ethanol (96%).

Formula

Ingredients	Quantity Required
Pilocarpine nitrate	0.1 g
Sodium chloride	0.068 g
Purified water q.s. to	10 ml

Apparatus

Glass beaker and measuring cylinder.

Procedure

Dissolve the sodium chloride in purified water, add pilocarpine nitrate and dissolve it by shaking. Makeup the volume 10 ml with purified water and sterilize the product by autoclaving.

Category

Antiglaucoma.

Dose

As directed by physician.

Therapeutic Use

It is used in the treatment of chronic open-angle glaucoma, acute angle-closure glaucoma, and ocular hypertension. It is also used to antagonize the effects of mydriasis and cycloplegia following surgery or ophthalmoscopic examination.

Storage

Pilocarpine Eye Drops BP should be stored in well-closed, light-resistant container in a cool place.

Label

'PROTECT FROM SUNLIGHT', 'FOR EXTERNAL USE ONLY' and 'NOT FOR INJECTION'.

Specimen Label

The specimen label for Pilocarpine Eye Drops BP is given as:

PILOCARPINE EYE DROPS BP **(10 ml)**		
Composition: Each 10 ml contains, Pilocarpine nitrate- 0.1 g Sodium chloride- 0.068 g Purified water q.s.- 10 ml **Dose:** As directed by physician. **Storage:** Store in well-closed, light-resistant container, in cool place.	**PILOCAR** (Eye Drops) (Used in glaucoma) **PROTECT FROM SUN LIGHT** **FOR EXTERNAL USE ONLY** **NOT FOR INJECTION** *(The contents should not be used for more than 1 month after the opening of container)*	**Mfg. Lic. No.-** 3D/2010 **Batch No.-** BH 812 **Mfg. Date-** Sep. 2011 **Exp. Date-** Aug. 2012 **M.R.P.-** Rs. 18.00 (Inclusive of all taxes) **Mfd. By:** GEET PHARMA JHANSI ROAD, GWALIOR, MP.

CHAPTER 17

NASAL PREPARATIONS

Nasal preparations are the formulations meant for instillation into the nasal cavities. These preparations may be of several categories like nasal drops and liquid nasal sprays, nasal powders, semisolid nasal preparations, nasal washes and nasal sticks. The first nasal solutions were formulated with menthol and thymol dissolved in light mineral oil. Later isotonic aqueous solutions were designed as drops.

Nasal preparations are supplied in single-dose or multi-dose containers provided, if necessary, with a suitable administration device which may be designed to avoid the introduction of contaminants. Aqueous nasal preparations supplied in multi-dose containers contain a suitable antimicrobial preservative in appropriate concentration, except where the preparation itself has adequate antimicrobial properties.

Nasal drops are solutions, emulsions or suspensions intended for instillation by means of a dropper or by spraying into the nasal cavities. They are usually buffered to pH of 6.8 and are isotonic with nasal secretions. These drops are used locally as antibiotics, anti-inflammatory, and decongestants. Nasal drops are the simplest and most convenient form. However, the exact volume of dosing is difficult to determine, which may be a device-related matter, and rapid drainage from the nose is another problem with drops.

Nasal drops that are solutions, should comply with the test of uniformity of mass. Weigh individually the contents of 10 containers emptied as completely as possible, and determine the average mass. Not more than 2 of the individual masses deviate by more than 10% from the average mass and none deviates by more than 20%.

Nasal drops that are emulsions, should have a uniform appearance after shaking and should not show evidence of phase separation. Suspensions should be readily redispersible on shaking to give a smooth and stable product. In suspensions, the size of the dispersed particles should be such as to localize their deposition in the nostril.

Oily solutions are not preferred since the oil may retard the ciliary action of the mucosa and may even cause lipoid pneumonia, if drop of oil enters the trachea. A vehicle for formulating nasal drops should have (a) pH between 5.5 and 7.5, (b) buffering capacity, (c) tonicity equivalent to normal saline, and (d) viscosity not exceeding the normal viscosity of nasal mucosa.

Nasal drops are supplied in 10 to 25 ml quantities in colored fluted bottles fitted with a screw cap and dropper, which is suitable for administration and avoids the introduction of contaminants.

Method of Preparation

Since nasal drops can be a simple solution, emulsion or suspension hence they can be prepared by their respective methods. Nasal drops are prepared using methods designed to avoid the introduction of contaminants and growth of microorganisms. During the development of a nasal preparation, the formulation for which contains an antimicrobial preservative, the effectiveness of the chosen preservative shall be demonstrated properly.

Therapeutic Uses

The use of nasal drops depends on the incorporated active ingredients. These are generally used for their antiseptic, local analgesic or vasoconstriction properties. Nasal drops may contain anti-inflammatory agents like corticosteroids, betamethasone, sympathomimetics like ephedrine hydrochloride and decongestants like phenylephrine, oxymetazoline, tetrahydrozoline hydrochloride to relieve nasal congestion.

Dose

Dose is prescribed on the basis of incorporated drug or as directed by physician.

Storage Conditions

Nasal drops should be stored in an airtight, tamper proof, sterile container to protect from microorganisms. Containers should be made from materials that do not cause deterioration of the preparation as a result of diffusion into or across the material of the container or by yielding foreign substances to the preparation. The container and package of a single dose preparation should be such as to maintain sterility of the contents and the applicator up to the time of use.

Containers for multiple application preparations should be fitted with an integral dropper or with a sterile screw cap of suitable materials incorporating a dropper and plastic or rubber teat. Alternatively, such a cap assembly may be packed separately after it is sterilized. Containers of multiple application preparations should permit the withdrawal of successive doses of the preparation.

Specific Labeling Requirement

The label of nasal drops should state (1) the names and concentrations in percentages, or weight or volume per ml of the active ingredients, (2) the names and concentrations of any added antimicrobial preservative, (3) the contents should not be used for more than 1 month after opening the container, (4) that the preparation is 'NOT FOR INJECTION', 'FOR EXTERNAL USE ONLY', and (5) the conditions under which the preparation should be stored.

Examples of Some Nasal Preparations

1. Phenylephrine Hydrochloride Nasal Drops

Phenylephrine hydrochloride is a frequent constituent of nasal decongestant preparations for topical use. It is a selective α_1 agonist, thus causes vasoconstriction. It is very sensitive to light and atmospheric oxygen hence undergoes oxidation. Therefore, sodium metabisulphite is used as antioxidant.

Composition	Method of Preparation
Phenylephrine hydrochloride- 0.23 g Sodium metabisulphite- 0.1 g Sodium chloride- 0.53 g Chlorbutol- 0.45 g Propylene glycol- 4.5 ml Purified water q.s.- 100 ml	Weigh accurately the chlorbutol, powder it and add in hot purified water (60°C) and quickly insert the stopper in conical flask to prevent its volatilization. Shake until solution completes. Cool the solution and add required quantity of phenylephrine hydrochloride, sodium metabisulphite, sodium chloride and propylene glycol, dissolve them by stirring, filter it and makeup the final volume with purified water and mix.

Label

PHENYLEPHRINE HYDROCHLORIDE NASAL DROPS (10 ml)		
Composition: Each 10 ml contains, Phenylephrine hydrochloride-0.023 g Chlorbutol- 0.045 g Purified water q.s.- 10 ml **Dose:** As directed by physician. **Storage:** Store in a well-closed, light-resistant container in a cool place.	**PHENRIDE** (Nasal Drops) (Used as a nasal decongestant) **PROTECT FROM SUN LIGHT** **FOR EXTERNAL USE ONLY** **NOT FOR INJECTION** *(The contents should not be used for more than 1 month after the opening of container)*	**Mfg. Lic. No.-** 2B/2010 **Batch No.-** KU 461 **Mfg. Date-** Sep. 2011 **Exp. Date-** Aug. 2012 **M.R.P.-** Rs. 15.00 (Inclusive of all taxes) **Mfd. By:** SOLEMN PHARMA HAMIDIA ROAD, BHOPAL, MP-462001

Marketed Preparations

Active Ingredient(s)	Marketed Preparation (Manufacturer)
Xylometazoline	**OTRIVIN** (NOVARTIS), **XYLOCHEK** (INDOCO), **XYBELV** (BLUBELL PHARMA), **DECON** (LE SANTE), **OTRITAL** (TALSON PHARMA)
Oxymetazoline	**METZOL** (SOLITAIRE), **NASIVION** (MERCK), **RHINOJET** (MERCK)
Phenylephrine	**DRISTRAN NASAL DROPS** (WYETH), **FENX NASAL DROPS** (ABBOTT)
Ephedrine	**ENDRIE** (WYETH)

EXERCISE - 29

Object

To prepare and submit 10 ml of Ephedrine Hydrochloride Nasal Drops BPC.

Principle

Nasal drops are liquid dosage forms, which are intended for instillation by means of a dropper or by spraying into the nasal cavities. They are usually buffered to pH 6.8 and are isotonic with nasal secretions.

The local application of Ephedrine Hydrochloride Nasal Drops BPC to the mucous membrane of the nose stimulates the vasoconstrictor sympathetic nerve endings hence reduces the nasal secretions. If the mucous membrane is inflamed, ephedrine relieves symptoms of painful swelling.

In this preparation ephedrine hydrochloride acts as nasal decongestant. Sodium chloride is used to make nasal drops isotonic with nasal secretions. Chlorbutol acts as a preservative.

Formula

Ingredients	Quantity Required
Ephedrine hydrochloride	0.05 g
Chlorbutol	0.05 g
Sodium chloride	0.05 g
Purified water q.s. to	10 ml

Apparatus

Glass beaker, conical flask and measuring cylinder.

Procedure

Weigh accurately the chlorbutol, powder it and add in hot purified water (60°C) and quickly insert the stopper in conical flask to prevent its volatilization. Shake until solution completes. Cool the solution and add ephedrine hydrochloride and sodium chloride, dissolve them by stirring, filter it and makeup the volume to 10 ml with purified water and mix.

Category

Nasal decongestant.

Dose

Two drops should be instilled into nostrils or as directed by physician.

Therapeutic Use

It is used as a nasal decongestant. It also relieves allergic and vasomotor rhinitis and sinusitis.

Storage

Ephedrine Hydrochloride Nasal Drops BPC should be stored in well-closed, light-resistant container in a cool place.

Label

'PROTECT FROM SUNLIGHT', 'NOT FOR INJECTION', 'FOR EXTERNAL USE ONLY'.

Specimen Label

The specimen label for Ephedrine Hydrochloride Nasal Drops BPC is given as:

<table>
<tr><td colspan="3">EPHEDRINE HYDROCHLORIDE NASAL DROPS BPC
(10 ml)</td></tr>
<tr>
<td>Composition:
Each 10 ml contains,
Ephedrine hydrochloride- 0.05 g
Chlorbutol- 0.05 g
Purified water q.s.- 10 ml
Dose: As directed by physician.
Storage: Store in a well closed, light-resistant container in a cool place.
(The contents should not be used for more than 1 month after the opening of container)</td>
<td>PHEDRIN
(Nasal Drops)
(Used as a nasal decongestant)

NOT FOR INJECTION
FOR EXTERNAL USE ONLY</td>
<td>Mfg. Lic. No.- 2H/2010
Batch No.- KA 212
Mfg. Date- July 2011
Exp. Date- June 2012

M.R.P.- Rs. 18.00
(Inclusive of all taxes)

Mfd. By: BETUL PHARMA BAROTIWALA ROAD, BADDI, SOLAN H.P.</td>
</tr>
</table>

CHAPTER 18

PILLS

Pills are small, solid masses of a globular, ovoid, or lenticular shape intended for oral administration. These usually range in weight from 0.10 to 0.30 g. Exceptionally large pills of 0.60 g or more are referred to as boluses and very small sugar-coated pills of 0.06 g or less are known as parvules or granules. The globules or orbicules are small spheres of sugar saturated with an alcoholic tincture, largely used in homeopathic medicine.

When the pill came into use in ancient Mesopotamia and Egypt, it offered for the first time a definite dose corresponding with a desired therapeutic action. The Greeks named the little balls of medicine *katapotia* (''something to be swallowed''), later Latinized to *catapotium*; by the first century A.D., the term *pilula* came into use in Rome.

Pills persisted as a major dosage form for a remarkably long period of time. Moreover, certain combinations of drugs persisted for thousands of years in pill form. The Pills of Rufus, for example, were originally a *hiera* (bitter powder) made into pill form by the Arabs and popularized by Avicenna (980-1033); a modern version, Pills of Aloe and Mastic, were last official in the 8th revision of the USP (1905).

Pills were the most common oral dose form in the nineteenth century for drugs with smaller volume doses. They were perceived to be relatively easy to make and compact in quantity, masked unpleasant tastes and odors, were stable for long periods and were easy to administer. It was only during the twentieth century that the poor bioavailability characteristics of pills as a dose form were discovered: pills were as likely to pass through the gastrointestinal tract unaltered as to disintegrate and deliver active ingredients, particularly when used in a coated form.

Method of Preparation

In order to prepare pills by hand, a pill base or mass is constructed from which the prescriber often directed that a given weight of mass should be made into a specified number of pills.

The pill mass is consisted of two parts: the active ingredients and the excipients, which provide the mass the appropriate consistency of adhesiveness, firmness and plasticity. Generally pills excipients contain glucose, glycerin, powdered acacia and benzoic acid.

The benzoic acid was often used as a preservative and might be omitted if only a small batch of pill mass was being compounded. The excipients formed a colorless, very adhesive liquid that was usually prepared in advance of compounding the pills. The active ingredients and excipient are triturated in a mortar with a special pill pestle and kneaded into a homogeneous mass that could be divided into the desired weight. The required weight of mass was then rolled into an elongated cylinder on a pill tile, which often incorporated a measuring scale to aid cutting and division.

Small quantities of mass were rolled using a pill spatula that had very little 'spring' and featured a broad end or a flat impervious board. The cylindrical pill mass was then cut either by hand or using a pill divider (a grooved roller) and then rolled into the final shape using a pill roller (resembling interlocking jar lids) or between the fingers.

Larger quantities of pills were generally made using a special pill machine. This consisted of two hardwood boards on which were mounted brass plates indented with hemispherical grooves (cutters). A cylindrical 'pipe' of pill mass would be laid across the grooves of the lower board. The upper and lower boards could be interfaced so that the grooves corresponded, and the upper board had handles which allowed the formulator to cut the mass into uniform pieces. Different sized pills could be cut by using different sized cutting plates.

Pills can be prevented from sticking to either the tile or the machine by use of a dusting powder such as rice flour. Pills were often coated with a variety of substances such as gold or silver leaf, gelatin or varnish (by treating with a solution of sandarac in ether and alcohol, which was allowed to evaporate), chocolate or keratin. The coating of pills effectively disguised unpleasant tastes and odors, rendered the pill more attractive and, in the case of precious metals, added to their therapeutic efficacy.

Commercially produced pills were often given a sugar or pearl (using finely powdered talcum or French chalk) coating, which was difficult to accomplish on a small scale.

Therapeutic Uses

The use of Pills depends on the corresponding use of incorporated active ingredients.

Dose

Dose is prescribed on the basis of incorporated drug or as directed by physician.

Storage Conditions

Pills are usually stored in a flat, circular or square box which was preferably made so shallow that the pills could not lie on top of one another. A light coating of dusting powder was included in the pill box to prevent freshly made pills adhering to each other.

Specific Labeling Requirement

The label of pills should state the names and concentrations of the active ingredients, the conditions under which the preparation should be stored. 'PROTECT FROM SUN LIGHT', 'KEEP IN COOL AND DRY PLACE'.

Examples of Some Pills

1. Aloe Pills

Composition	Method of Preparation
Aloe- 0.18 g Excipient q.s.- 2 g	Incorporate aloe with other excipients to form a cohesive, plastic mass, which is divided into 10 portions, each of which is formed into the desired round shape.

<table>
<tr><td colspan="3" align="center">Label</td></tr>
<tr><td colspan="3" align="center">ALOE PILLS
(10 Pills)</td></tr>
<tr>
<td>Composition:
Each 10 Pills contains,
Aloe- 0.18 g
Excipient q.s.- 2 g
Dose: As directed by physician.
Storage: Store in a well-closed, light-resistant container in a cool place.</td>
<td align="center">ALOVI
(Pills)

(Used as purgative)

PROTECT FROM SUN LIGHT</td>
<td>Mfg. Lic. No.- 2M/2010
Batch No.- VG 213
Mfg. Date- Mar. 2011
Exp. Date- Feb. 2012
M.R.P.- Rs. 11.00
(Inclusive of all taxes)
Mfd. By: TANVI PHARMA JHANSI ROAD, BHOPAL, M.P.- 462001</td>
</tr>
</table>

2. Belladonna Opium Pills

Composition	Method of Preparation
Belladonna extract- 0.030 g Opium (powder)- 0.030 g Excipients q.s.- 1 g	Incorporate belladonna extract and opium with other excipients to form a cohesive, plastic mass, divide into 10 portions, each of which is formed into the desired round shape.

<table>
<tr><td colspan="3" align="center">**Label**</td></tr>
</table>

BELLADONNA OPIUM PILLS **(10 Pills)**		
Composition: Each 10 Pills contains, Belladonna extract- 0.030 g Opium (powder)- 0.030 g Excipients q.s.- 1 g **Dose:** As directed by physician. **Storage:** Store in well-closed container in a cool place.	**BELLOPI** (Pills) (Used as a sedative) **PROTECT FROM SUN LIGHT**	**Mfg. Lic. No.-** 4F/2010 **Batch No.-** CH 184 **Mfg. Date-** Aug. 2011 **Exp. Date-** July 2012 **M.R.P.-** Rs. 18.00 (Inclusive of all taxes) **Mfd. By:** YANA PHARMACEUTICALS INDUSTRIAL AREA, SONEPAT, HARYANA- 131001

Marketed Preparations

Several Homeopathic preparations are marketed in the form of Pills.

EXERCISE - 30

Object

To prepare and submit 10 pills of Ipecac.

Principle

Pill is an ancient dosage form of presenting solid medication. Generally pills excipients contain glucose, glycerin, powdered acacia and benzoic acid. Pills can be prevented from sticking to either the tile or the machine by use of a dusting powder such as rice flour. Pills are usually stored in a flat, circular or square box which was preferably made so shallow that the pills could not lie on top of one another.

Formula

Ingredients	Quantity Required
Calomel	0.01 g
Ipecac (powder)	1 g

Apparatus

Glass beaker, measuring cylinder and pill board.

Procedure

Pills are made by mixing the calomel and ipecac powder with an excipient in a mortar and pestle to form a paste, then rolling the mass into a long cylindrical shape (called a "pipe"), and dividing it into equal 10 portions, which are then rolled into rounded pills.

Category

Expectorant.

Dose

As directed by physician.

Therapeutic Use

It is used as stimulant expectorant.

Storage

Ipecac pills should be stored in well-closed, light-resistant container in a cool and dry place.

Label

'PROTECT FROM SUNLIGHT'.

Specimen Label

The specimen label for Ipecac Pills is given as:

<table>
<tr><td colspan="3" align="center">IPECAC PILLS
(10 Pills)</td></tr>
<tr>
<td>Composition:
Each 10 Pills contains,
Calomel- 0.01 g
Ipecac (powder) q.s.- 1 g
Dose: As directed by physician.
Storage: Store in well-closed, light-resistant container in a cool and dry place.</td>
<td align="center">PILOCAR
(Pills)

(Used as a stimulant expectorant)

PROTECT FROM SUN LIGHT</td>
<td>Mfg. Lic. No.- 3D/2010
Batch No.- BH 812
Mfg. Date- Sep. 2011
Exp. Date- Aug. 2012
M.R.P.- Rs. 18.00
(Inclusive of all taxes)
Mfd. By: YAVI PHARMA
KANPUR ROAD,
LUCKNOW UP- 226001</td>
</tr>
</table>

CHAPTER 19

LOZENGES

Lozenges are unit solid dosages forms containing medicament in a sweetened and flavored base, intended to dissolve slowly in the mouth. A throat lozenge is a small, medicated, sweet intended to be dissolved slowly in the mouth to temporarily stop coughs and lubricate and soothe irritated tissues of the throat (usually due to a sore throat), possibly from the common cold or influenza. These are mainly used for prolonged action of the medicament on the throat, and to medicate the mouth and throat. Along with the medicament these usually consist of sugar, flavoring agent and a strong binding agent. The binding agent provides suitable hardness, cohesiveness and slow release of the medicament. Due to the presence of binding agent, lozenges do not disintegrate in the mouth but dissolve slowly and release the active medicaments. High contents of sugar and gum produce a sticky solution in the mouth that causes the medicament to adhere on the affected surface of the throat.

Lozenges may contain benzocaine, an anesthetic, or eucalyptus oil. Non-menthol throat lozenges generally use either zinc gluconate, glycine or pectin as an oral demulcent. Several preparations of throat lozenges contain dextromethorphan. Still other varieties contain menthol, peppermint oil or spearmint as their active ingredient. Honey lozenges are also available.

Method of Preparation

Lozenges are prepared by two methods: Moulding method (moulded lozenges) and Compression method (compressed lozenges).

(a) Moulding Method

It is a traditional and most widely used method of preparation of lozenges. The most important step in this method is the formation of lozenge mass which is made up of medicament, powdered sucrose, gum and water. In certain cases inert substance like starch or dextrose is used to provide suitable body to the lozenges. The composition of simple mass is as follows-

207

Ingredients	Method of Preparation
Sucrose (fine powder)- 100 g Acacia (fine powder)- 7 g Purified water- q.s.	Take the required quantity of sucrose and acacia in a mortar and add purified water in small proportions until dough like mass is formed by kneading. Kneading should be continued until mass tends to be soft enough.

After the preparation of soft mass, weigh the mass to determine the weight and size of the finished lozenges. For rolling the mass lozenge board and roller is used. During the rolling, board and roller should be dusted with starch, lactose or talc to prevent the sticking. Mass is rolled on the board to get the uniform thickness. Cut the lozenges by the punches of specific shape and place them on a perforated tray dusted over with starch or talc and dry for 24 hours in hot air oven at 40°C to obtain uniform hardness.

(b) Compression Method

In this method lozenges are prepared by tablet compression machine with some modifications like use of high compression, no addition of disintegrant and incorporation of high percentage of binding agent (usually more than 50% of sucrose and gum acacia or tragacanth). In this method drug, sucrose and binding agent are mixed together with water to make damp mass which is passed through a sieve to obtain the granules. These granules are dried and compressed into the lozenges.

Some medicaments are deteriorated by moisture and temperature hence in such cases lozenges are prepared by compressing the mixture of medicament with previously prepared and dried granules of sucrose or lactose. To prevent the volatilization of flavoring agents, they are added after granulation.

Therapeutic Uses

The use of lozenges depends on the corresponding use of incorporated active ingredients. Generally these are used as expectorant and demulcent in the treatment of cough and as mild antiseptic in sore throat.

Dose

One lozenge to be sucked slowly at definite time interval as directed by physician.

Storage Conditions

Lozenges should be stored in air tight containers in a cool and dry place as they become soft in damp conditions.

Specific Labeling Requirement

The label of lozenge should state (1) the names and concentrations of the active ingredients, (2) the conditions under which the preparation should be stored, and (3) 'DO NOT SWALLOW'.

Examples of Some Lozenges

1. Compound Bismuth Lozenges BPC

Bismuth carbonate works as antidiarrheal agent. Calcium carbonate and heavy magnesium carbonate act as antacids.

Composition	Method of Preparation
Calcium carbonate- 1.5 g Bismuth carbonate- 3 g Heavy magnesium carbonate- 1.5 g Rose oil- q.s. Simple base q.s.- 10 g	These lozenges are prepared by Moulding method. Accurately weigh the ingredients and mix uniformly in a mortar, add simple base and knead to produce a mass of required consistency then mix the rose oil. Dust the lozenge board and roller with starch, lactose or talc to prevent the sticking. Mass is rolled on the board to get uniform thickness then cut the lozenges by the punches of specific shape. After cutting place the lozenges on a perforated tray dusted over with starch or talc and dry for 24 hours in hot air oven at 40°C to obtain uniform hardness.

Label

COMPOUND BISMUTH LOZENGES BPC **(10 Lozenges)**		
Composition: Each lozenge contains, Calcium carbonate-0.15 g Bismuth carbonate- 0.3 g Heavy magnesium carbonate- 0.15 g Simple base q.s.- 1 g **Dose:** One lozenge should be sucked slowly every 4 hours. **Storage:** Store in a well-closed, container in a dry place.	**COMBIS** (Lozenges) (Used as antidiarrhoeal and antacid) **DO NOT SWALLOW**	**Mfg. Lic. No.-** 3H/2010 **Batch No.-** KS 912 **Mfg. Date-** June 2011 **Exp. Date-** May 2012 **M.R.P.-** Rs. 15.00 (Inclusive of all taxes) **Mfd. By:** YAVI PHARMA KANPUR ROAD, LUCKNOW UP- 226001

2. Cetylpyridinium Chloride Lozenges USP

Benzocaine is a mild local anaesthetic. Cetylpyridinium chloride is quarternary pyridinium antiseptic compound. It has antibacterial and antifungal properties. Some Gram-negative bacteria, especially *Pseudomonas cepacia*, are resistant. Benzocaine is contraindicated in patients with low plasma-cholinesterase concentrations or in those receiving anticholinesterases. It is not recommended for children under 6 years of age.

Composition	Method of Preparation
Cetylpyridinium chloride- 0.015 g Benzocaine- 0.12 g Simple base q.s.- 1 g	These lozenges are prepared by Moulding method. Accurately weigh the ingredients and mix uniformly in a mortar, add simple base and knead to produce a mass of required consistency. Dust the lozenge board and roller with starch, lactose or talc to prevent the sticking. Mass is rolled on the board to get uniform thickness then cut the lozenges by the punches of specific shape. After cutting, place the lozenges on a perforated tray dusted over with starch or talc and dry for 24 hours in hot air oven at 40°C to obtain uniform hardness.

Label

<table>
<tr><td colspan="3" align="center">CETYLPYRIDINIUM CHLORIDE LOZENGES USP
(10 Lozenges)</td></tr>
<tr>
<td>Composition:
Each lozenge contains,
Cetylpyridinium chloride- 0.015 g
Benzocaine- 0.12 g
Simple base q.s.- 1 g
Dose: One lozenge should be sucked slowly every 2-3 hours.
Storage: Store in well-closed container in a cool place.</td>
<td align="center">CETORIDE
(Lozenges)
(Used for symptomatic relief of sore throat)

PROTECT FROM SUN LIGHT
KEEP OUT OF REACH OF CHILDREN
DO NOT SWALLOW</td>
<td>Mfg. Lic. No.- 2B/2010
Batch No.- FH 264
Mfg. Date- Sep. 2011
Exp. Date- Aug. 2012
M.R.P.- Rs. 19.00
(Inclusive of all taxes)
Mfd. By: YANA PHARMA KALPI ROAD, KANPUR, U.P.</td>
</tr>
</table>

Marketed Preparations

Active Ingredient(s)	Marketed Preparation (Manufacturer)
Dextromethorphan HBr	**ALEX COUGH LOZENGES** (GRACEWELL)
Noscapine	**CHERANA COUGH LOZENGES** (KNOLL PHARMA)
Dequalinium chloride	**DEQUADIN** (WELLCOME)
Ginger and Lemon	**COFSITS** (CIPLA)
Dichlorobenzyl alcohol and Amylmetacresol	**STREPSILS** (BOOTS LTD.)

EXERCISE - 31

Object

To prepare and submit 10 Liquorice Lozenges (Brompton Cough Lozenges) BPC.

Principle

Lozenges are solid preparations that are intended to dissolve or disintegrate slowly in the mouth to obtain, usually, a local effect in the oral cavity and the throat.

The extract of liquorice is prepared by the dried roots and stolons of *Glycyrrhiza glabra*. It consists of triterpenoid saponin, known as glycyrrhizin which acts as expectorant and demulscent.

Formula

Ingredients	Quantity Required
Liquorice extract	0.24 g
Anise oil	0.03 ml
Simple base q.s. to	1 g

Apparatus

Glass beaker, measuring cylinder, lozenge board and roller.

Procedure

These lozenges are prepared by Moulding method. Mix the required quantity of liquorice extract and anise oil uniformly in a mortar, add simple base and knead to produce a mass of required consistency. Dust the lozenge board and roller with starch, lactose or talc to prevent the sticking. Mass is rolled on the board to get uniform thickness then cut the lozenges by the punches of specific shape. After cutting place the lozenges on a perforated tray dusted over with starch or talc and dry for 24 hours in hot air oven at 40°C to obtain uniform hardness.

Category

Expectorant.

Dose

One lozenge should be sucked slowly at every 1 hour or as directed by physician.

Therapeutic Use

It is used as expectorant and demulcent for the treatment of cough.

Storage

Liquorice Lozenges BPC should be stored in well closed container in a cool and dry place at room temperature not exceeding 25°C.

Label

'PROTECT FROM SUNLIGHT', 'DO NOT SWALLOW'.

Specimen Label

The specimen label for Liquorice Lozenges (Brompton Cough Lozenges) BPC is given as:

<table>
<tr><td colspan="3" align="center">LIQUORICE LOZENGES BPC
(10 Lozenges)</td></tr>
<tr>
<td>

Composition:

Each lozenge contains,

Liquorice extract- 0. 24 g

Anise oil- 0.03 ml

Simple base q.s.- 1g

Dose: One lozenge should be sucked slowly every 1 hour.

Storage: Store in well-closed, container in a dry place.

</td>
<td align="center">

LIQLOZ

(Lozenges)

(Used as expectorant)

PROTECT FROM SUN LIGHT

DO NOT SWALLOW

</td>
<td>

Mfg. Lic. No.- 2J/2010

Batch No.- CN 612

Mfg. Date- May 2011

Exp. Date- April 2012

M.R.P.- Rs. 14.00

(Inclusive of all taxes)

Mfd. By: YAVI PHARMA

KANPUR ROAD,

LUCKNOW UP- 226001

</td>
</tr>
</table>

CHAPTER 20

PASTILLES

Pastilles are solid, single-dose preparations intended to dissolve in mouth to obtain, usually, a local effect in the oral cavity and the throat. They contain one or more active substances, usually in a flavored and sweetened base, and are intended to dissolve or disintegrate slowly in the mouth when sucked. Pastilles are soft, flexible preparations prepared by moulding of mixtures containing natural or synthetic polymers or gums and sweeteners.

Pastilles are a form of lozenge, particularly those which are chocolate flavored; also, combustible cones of aromatic drugs used for fumigation. The term came into english usage around 1650 from the French pastille, which was derived from the Latin *pastillus*, meaning ''little loaf''.

Pastilles were originally a pill shaped lump of compressed herbs, which was burnt to release its medicinal properties. They were also widely used during the eighteenth century in Western cultures to take herbal curatives and medicines, which eventually were developed into candies.

Pastilles are a type of candy or medicinal pill made of a thick liquid that has been solidified and is meant to be consumed by light chewing and allowing it to dissolve in the mouth. They are also used to describe certain forms of incense. A pastille is also known as a "troche", or a medicated lozenge that dissolves like candy.

Pastilles are made by pouring thick liquids into a powdered, sugared, or waxed mold and then allowing the liquid to set and dry. The substances contained in the dried liquid are slowly released when chewed and allowed to dissolve in the mouth. The substances are then absorbed by the mucous membranes of the oral cavity or in the lower gastro-intestinal tracts. Various substances of medicinal nature or for flavor can be put into pastille forms.

Due to the oily nature of these active substances (essential oils, tinctures and extracts), pastilles are usually based on a mixture of starch and gum arabic, which emulsifies the substance and binds them in a hydrocolloidal matrix. The starch and gum also reduce the rate in which the pastille dissolves and moderates the amount of active substances delivered at a time. Gum arabic also hardens the pastilles and makes them sturdier in storage and transport.

Only two pastilles are official in BPC i.e. Squill Pastilles and Opiate Pastilles (Gee's Pastilles).

Method of Preparation:

Pastilles are prepared by incorporating the medicament in suitable pastilles base. Since the medicament is intended to have a prolonged local action, the base should be firm enough to ensure that the pastilles should dissolve slowly. Generally gelatin or glycerol-gelatin base is used. The compositions of glycerol-gelatin base with its modifications are given below:

(a) For soft base

Ingredients	Quantity Required
Gelatin	1 part
Glycerin	2.5 parts
Purified water	2.5 parts

(b) For firm base

Ingredients	Quantity Required
Gelatin	30 parts
Glycerin	75 parts
Acacia	8 parts
Aromatic water	60 parts

(c) For hard base

Ingredients	Quantity Required
Acacia	18 parts
Sugar	6 parts
Purified water	80 parts

Due to the high gelatin content in glycerol-gelatin, pastilles produce a sticky solution in the mouth than lozenges. This property is advantageous when a local action like antiseptic or anesthetic effect is required in the mouth or throat.

Pastilles are prepared by moulding method using metallic mould of specific shape and size. The mould consists of a number of saucer shaped cavities. For the preparation of pastilles, soften the gelatin with hot water and add glycerin, stir until a clear solution is obtained. Add the medicament to the glycerol-gelatin solution, just before the solution gets stiffen and stir until the mass become homogeneous and firm enough. Lubricate the cavities of mould by liquid paraffin and pour the melted base into the cavities of mould up to the brim to ensure the uniformity in size. After cooling, dry the prepared pastilles by spreading them on a sheet of butter paper.

Note :

(a) Since the quantity of medicament in pastilles is usually small, hence there is no need to calculate the displacement value of the medicament.

(b) If alkaloidal salts are present then they should be dissolved in a small quantity of water, before adding to the base to ensure their uniform distribution.

Therapeutic Uses

The use of pastilles depends on the corresponding use of incorporated active ingredients. Generally these are used as expectorant and demulcent in the treatment of cough. These are also used for minor throat and bronchial irritation occurring with the common cold or inhaled irritants or sore throat.

Dose

One pastille should be sucked slowly at every definite period of time or as directed by physician.

Storage Conditions

Pastilles should be stored in well closed containers in a cool and dry place or at room temperature, not exceeding 25°C.

Specific Labeling Requirement

The label of pastilles should state (1) the names and concentrations of the active ingredients, (2) the directions for use of the pastilles, (3) the date after which the pastilles are not intended to be used, and (4) the conditions under which they should be stored.

Examples of Some Pastilles

1. Menthol and Eucalyptus oil Pastilles

Menthol is the main constituent of peppermint oil which is obtained from plant *Mentha piperita*. Menthol acts as antiseptic, stimulant, counter irritant and flavoring agent. Eucalyptus oil is obtained from leaves of *Eucalyptus globules*. It consists mainly eucalyptol which acts as antiseptic, expectorant and counter irritant.

Composition	Method of Preparation
Menthol- 0.003 g Eucalyptus oil- 0.03 ml Glycero-gelatin base q.s.- 2 g	Dissolve the menthol in eucalyptus oil and add to the melted glycero-gelatin base and mix uniformly. Pour the hot mass into the cavities of the lubricated mould and allow it to cool. After cooling, inverse the mould on a sheet of butter paper to collect the pastilles.

Label

MENTHOL AND EUCALYPTUS OIL PASTILLES (10 Pastilles)		
Composition: Each pastille contains, Menthol- 0.003 g Eucalyptus oil- 0.03 ml Glycero-gelatin base q.s.- 2 g **Dose:** One pastille should be sucked slowly every 4 hour. **Storage:** Store in a well- closed container, in a cool place.	**MENTHOTUS** (Pastilles) (Used as expectorant and demulcent) **DO NOT SWALLOW PROTECT FROM SUN LIGHT**	**Mfg. Lic. No.-** 6H/2010 **Batch No.-** DG 712 **Mfg. Date-** Jun 2011 **Exp. Date-** May 2012 **M.R.P.-** Rs. 14.00 (Inclusive of all taxes) **Mfd. By:** YASH PHARMACEUTICALS SITAPUR ROAD, LUCKNOW UP- 226001

Marketed Preparations

No marketed preparation is available.

EXERCISE - 32

Object

To prepare and submit 10 Ammonium Chloride Pastilles.

Principle

Pastille is a solid oral preparation consisting of one or more medicaments in an inert base and intended to dissolve slowly in the mouth. Ammonium chloride acts as expectorant. These pastilles are made up of soft base i.e. Glycero-gelatin base. Gelatin dissolves in hot water and forms solution, which on cooling sets as a jelly. This property of gelatin is utilized to convert glycerin into a solid form, to use as pastilles base. Glycerin is used as preservative to prevent the deterioration of gelatin. It also acts as non volatile hygroscopic emollient. These pastilles are prepared by moulding method using 2 g capacity mould.

Formula

(a) For Glycero-gelatin pastilles base

Ingredients	Quantity Required
Gelatin	1 g
Glycerin	2.5 ml
Purified water	2.5 ml

(b) For the preparation of pastilles

Ingredients	Quantity Required
Ammonium chloride	0.06 g
Liquid extract of liquorice	0.06 ml
Glycero-gelatin base q.s.	2 g

Apparatus

Glass beaker, measuring cylinder, china dish and water bath.

Procedure

Heat the glycerin at 100°C in a covered china dish on a water bath. Heat the purified water to boiling and add to the weighed quantity of gelatin, stir gently to dissolve. Add the hot glycerin to the aqueous solution of gelatin. Stir the mixture gently to avoid the entrapment of air bubbles until gel is formed. Maintain the base at 100°C for 1 hour to eliminate the microbial contaminants. Add the required quantity of ammonium chloride and liquid extract of liquorice and mix uniformly. Pour the hot mass into the cavities of the lubricated mould and allow it to cool. After cooling, inverse the mould on a sheet of butter paper to collect the pastilles.

Category

Expectorant Pastille.

Dose

One pastille should be sucked slowly, 5-6 pastilles per day or as directed by physician.

Therapeutic Use

These pastilles are used as expectorant and demulcent in the treatment of cough.

Storage

Ammonium chloride pastilles should be stored in well closed container in a cool place at room temperature not exceeding 25°C.

Label

'PROTECT FROM SUNLIGHT', 'DO NOT SWALLOW'.

Specimen Label

The specimen label for Ammonium Chloride Pastilles is given as:

<table>
<tr><td colspan="3" align="center">AMMONIUM CHLORIDE PASTILLES
(10 Pastilles)</td></tr>
<tr>
<td>Composition:
Each Pastille contains,
Ammonium chloride- 0.06 g
Liquid extract of liquorice- 0.06 ml
Glycero-gelatin base q.s.- 2 g
Dose: As directed by physician.
Storage: Store in well-closed container in dry place at temperature below 25°C.</td>
<td align="center">AMCHLO
(Pastilles)
(Used as expectorant)

PROTECT FROM SUN LIGHT
DO NOT SWALLOW</td>
<td>Mfg. Lic. No.- 2M/2010
Batch No.- VJ 512
Mfg. Date- Oct. 2011
Exp. Date- Sep. 2012
M.R.P.- Rs. 15.00
(Inclusive of all taxes)
Mfd. By: RAVI PHARMA
GWALIOR ROAD, JHANSI
UP- 284301</td>
</tr>
</table>

CHAPTER 21

SIZE REDUCTION

Many solid materials exist in sizes that are too large to be used directly in pharmaceutical preparations. Thus such materials must be reduced in suitable size. Size reduction may be defined as the process of reducing the size of a substance to a finer state of subdivision. It is a mechanical process of breakdown of solids into smaller size particles without altering the state of aggregation of solids. Grinding, Comminution or Milling are other terms used to signify size reduction. Size reduction of a drug may include one or more of the operations like cutting, slicing, chopping, pulverizing, micronizing etc.

Importance of Size Reduction

1. Mixing
2. Surface area
3. Drying
4. Effect on absorption
5. Color and texture
6. Effect on viscosity
7. Extraction
8. Smooth Appearance
9. Enhanced Stability
10. Less Irritation

Mechanism of Size Reduction

There are four main methods of size reduction, involving different mechanisms:

1. Cutting

The material is cut by means of sharp blades.

2. Compression

In this method the material is crushed by application of pressure.

3. Impact

Impact occurs when the material is more or less stationary and is hit by an object moving at high speed or when the moving particle strikes a stationary surface. Usually both will take place, since the substance is hit by a moving hammer and the particles formed are then thrown against the casing of the machine.

4. Attrition

In this method the material is subjected to pressure as in compression, but the surfaces are moving relative to each other, resulting in shear forces which break the particles.

Criteria for Selection of a Mill

(a) Product specifications

(b) Mill specifications

(c) Versatility of operation

(d) Dust control

(e) Sanitation

(f) Auxiliary equipments

(g) Mode of operation

(h) Economical factors

Ball Mill

A ball mill is an example of a comminution method which produces size reduction by both impact and attrition of particles.

The ball mill (Fig. 1) consists of a hollow cylinder mounted in such a way that it can be rotated on its horizontal longitudinal axis. The ball mill has length slightly greater than its diameter. Cylinder diameters can be greater than 3 meter, although much smaller sizes are used pharmaceutically. The cylinder may be of metal, porcelain or of rubber, to reduce abrasion. The mill is partially filled with balls which act as the grinding medium. The balls may be of metal or porcelain. The cylinder contains balls that occupy 30 to 50% of the mill volume, the ball size being dependent on the size of the feed and the diameter of the mill.

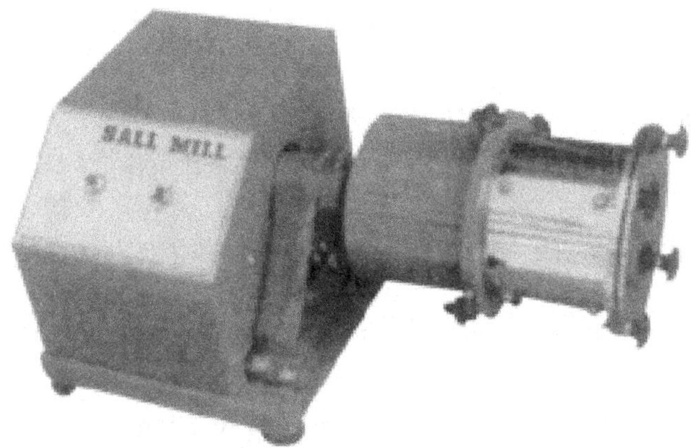

Fig. 1 Ball Mill

Note: For details the readers may refer to, "*A Text Book of Professional Pharmacy*", by Jain N. K. and Sharma S. N., Vallabh Prakashan, Delhi.

EXERCISE - 33

Object

To determine the effect of size of balls, number of balls and time on the efficiency of ball mill.

Theory

Milling (size reduction) is the mechanical process of reducing the particle size of solids. Various terms (crushing, disintegration, grinding and pulverization) have been used synonymously with comminution depending on the product, the equipment and the process. The surface area per unit weight (specific surface) is increased by size reduction which affects the therapeutic efficacy of medicinal substances.

A ball mill is a horizontal cylinder partly filled with steel balls (or occasionally other shapes) that rotates on its axis, imparting a tumbling and cascading action to the balls. Material fed through the mill is crushed by impact and ground by attrition between the balls.

Effect of Size of Balls

For a given feed smaller balls give a slower but a final grinding. The smaller balls provide smaller voids then the larger voids; consequently, the void through which material will flow without being struck by a ball is less and the no of impacts per unit weight of material is greater. The optimum diameter of a ball is proportional to the square root of the size of the feed:

$$D_{ball}^{2} = kD$$

where D_{ball} and D are the diameters of the ball and the feed particles respectively.

Effect of Number of Balls

Increasing the total weight of balls of a given size increases the fineness of powder the weight of ball charge can be increased by increasing the no balls and in other way by using a ball composed of a material with a higher density.

The optimum milling conditions are usually obtained when the bulk volume of the balls is equal to 50% of volume of the mill, variation in weight of balls is normally affected by the use of materials of different densities. Thus steel balls grind faster than porcelain balls.

Effect of Time

If the size of the balls and the number of balls are kept constant then by increasing the time the efficiency of the ball mill will increase as it produces more fine particles.

From the view point of power consumption wet grinding is more efficient then dry grinding. A slower speed is used in wet milling then in dry milling to prevent the mass from being carried around with the mill. Wetting agents may increase the efficiency of mill and the physical stability of the product by nullifying electrostatic forces produces during comminution.

Procedure

Take accurately weighed (100 g) of any dried crude drug and operate the ball mill having the same size and number of the balls for 15, 30, 45 minutes. The powdered drug is put in a set of sieves (#10, 36 and 60) and put on a sieve shaker for about 10 minute. The amount retained on each mesh is noted by weighing of individual powder. Finally find out the percentage amount retained on each sieve and calculate the effect of time on milling efficiency of the ball mill.

The similar procedure is repeated by keeping the time and number of balls constant but of different size of balls and finding out the percentage amount of powdered drug retained on each sieve to calculate the effect of size on the milling efficiency of the ball mill.

Further, to study the effect of the number of balls on milling efficiency of ball mill the size and time of milling is kept constant and the above procedure is repeated to calculate the amount of powder retained on each mesh.

Observation Table

Number of balls

Time of rotation

Initial weight of crude drug (g)	Weight after sieving through sieve # 10	Weight after sieving through sieve # 36	Weight after sieving through sieve # 60

Calculation

Sieve No.	Arithmetic mean size opening (μm)	Weight retained (g)	% retained on sieve	Weight size	Particle Size (μm)

Result

1. As the number of balls in Ball mill is increased, the size reduction increases.
2. As the size of the balls is increased, the size reduction decreases.
3. As the time is increased the size reduction increases.

CHAPTER 22

MIXING OF SOLIDS

Mixing is an operation in which two or more ingredients in separate or roughly mixed condition are treated so that each particle of any one ingredient is as nearly as possible adjacent to a particle of each of the other ingredients.

Objective

1. To secure uniformity of composition so that small samples withdrawn from a bulk material represent the overall composition of the mixture.
2. To promote physical or chemical reactions, such as dissolution, in which natural diffusion is supplemented by agitation.

Factors Influencing the Mixing of Powders

1. Volume of Material/Mixer
2. Handling of Mixed Powder
3. Duration of Mixing
4. Mixing Mechanism
5. Physical Properties of the Ingredients
   (a) Particle Attraction
   (b) Proportion of Mixing Materials
   (c) Particle Size and Shape
   (d) Density

Mechanisms of Mixing of Powders

1. Convective mixing
2. Shear mixing
3. Diffusive mixing

224

Equipments Used for Mixing

The ideal mixer should rapidly produce a complete blend with as gentle as possible a mixing action to avoid damage. It should be easily cleaned and discharged, be dust-tight, require low maintenance and low power consumption.

(a) Agitated Powder Mixers:

Agitator mixer depends on the motion of a blade or paddle through the product, and hence the main mixing mechanism is convection. Examples include the ribbon mixer and the Nauta Mixer.

1. Ribbon Mixer

A ribbon mixer (fixed-shell mixer or agitator mixer) consists of a relatively long through like shell with a semicircular bottom (Fig. 1).

In ribbon mixer, mixing is achieved by the rotation of helical blades in a hemispherical trough. 'Dead spots' are difficult to eliminate in this type of mixer and the shearing action caused by the movement of the blades may be insufficient to break up drug aggregates. The mixer does, however, mix poorly flowing material and is less likely to cause segregation than a tumbling mixer.

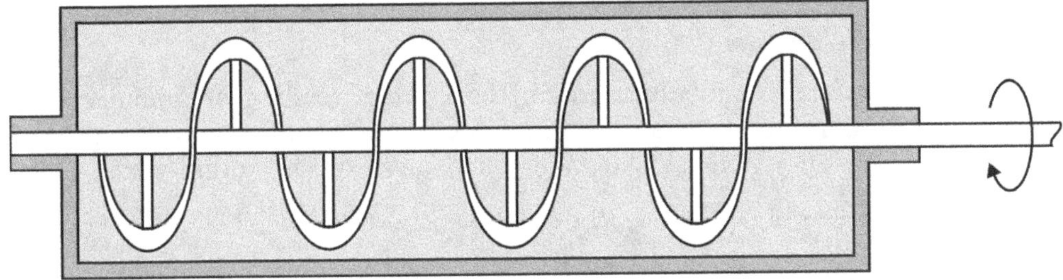

Fig. 1 Ribbon agitator powder mixer

2. Nauta Mixer

A more recent type of agitator mixer is the Nauta mixer (Fig. 2) that consists of a conical vessel fitted at the base with a rotating screw fastened to the end of a rotating arm at the top. The screw conveys material toward the top where it cascades back into the mass. The mixer thus combines convective mixing (as the material is raised by the helical conveyor) and shear and diffusive mixing (as the material cascades downwards).

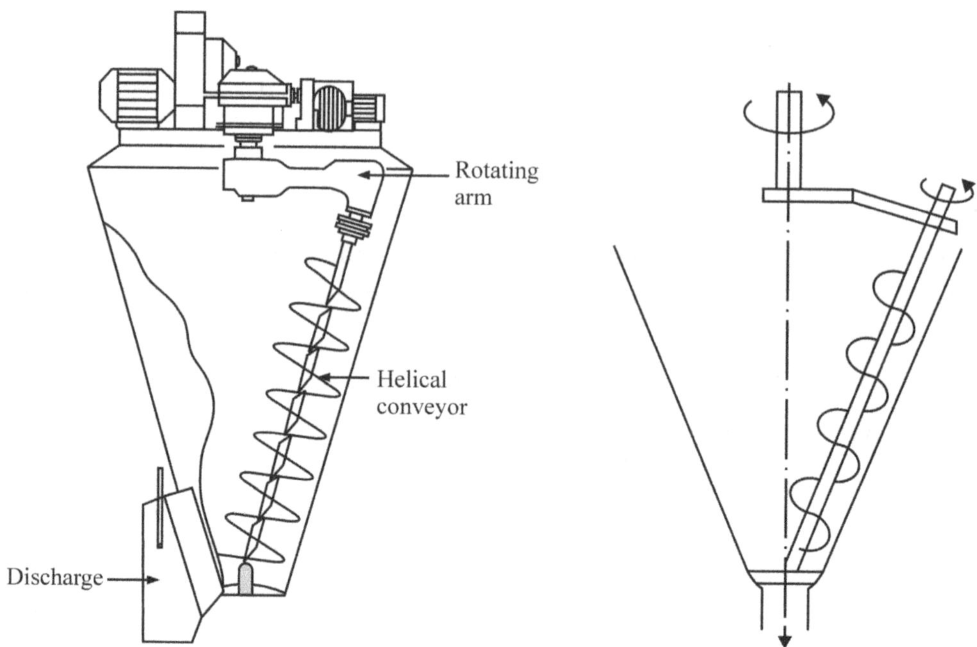

Fig. 2 Nauta mixer

(b) Tumbling Mixers/Blenders

Tumbling mixers are commonly used for the mixing/blending of granules or free-flowing powders. There are many different designs of tumbling mixer, e.g. double-cone mixers, twin-shell mixers, cube mixers, Y-cone mixers and drum mixers (Fig. 3).

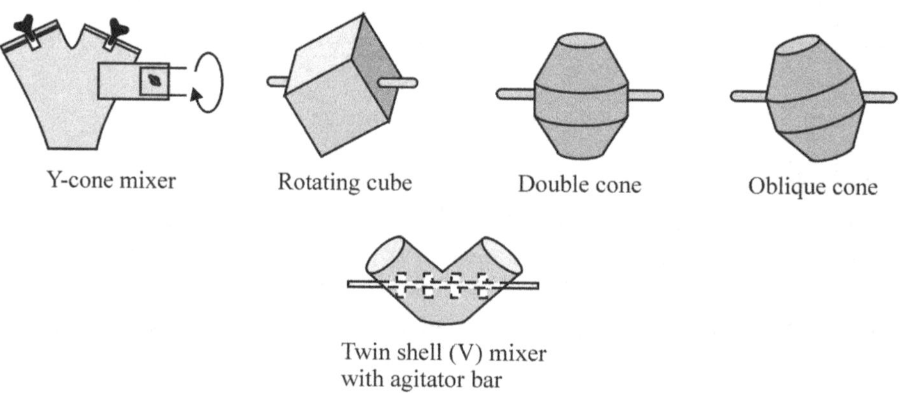

Fig. 3 Different designs of the tumbling mixers

Note: For details the readers may refer to, "*A Text Book of Professional Pharmacy*", by Jain N. K. and Sharma S. N., Vallabh Prakashan, Delhi.

EXERCISE - 34

Object

To determine the mixing efficiency of solid-solid mixing.

Theory

Solid-solid mixing is a process in which two or more than two solid substances are intermingled in a mixer by continuous movement of the particles. Mainly the object of mixing operation is to produce a bulk mixture which when divided in different doses every unit of dose must contain the correct proportion of each ingredient.

Batch Mixing

A common type of mixer consists of container of one or several geometric forms which is mounted so that it can be rotated about an axis. The popular twin cell blender is of this type and takes the form of a cylinder that has been cut in half at 45 degree angle with it's long axis and then rejoined to form a V shape this is rotated so that alternately collected in the bottom of V and then split into two portions when the V is inverted. This is quite effective.

Powder Mixing

In solid-solid mixing four steps are involved-

1. Expansion of bed of solid
2. Application of three dimensional shear forces to the powder bed
3. Mix long enough to permit true randomization of particles
4. Maintain randomization (No segregation after mixing)

Procedure

To estimate the efficiency of solid-solid mixing using a common type of mixer, two materials (e.g. brick powder and oxalic acid) may be selected in which one is inert powder. The weighed quantities of these two drugs are put in the mixer and allow the mixing operation for a certain period of time at particular speed. After a specified time, the powdered sample is taken out randomly from different places of mixer and the amount of active drug present is calculated on the basis of titration method. The same procedure will be repeated by differing the speed of mixer so that the effect of speed of rotation of mixer can be determined.

The efficiency of solid-solid mixing (Mixing Index) can be calculated by following steps

1. Prepare the standard solution of oxalic acid and standardized sodium hydroxide solution by standard oxalic acid.

2. Mix the brick powder and oxalic acid in a given ratio and put in twin blade mixer and mixed for 5 minutes.

3. Take 5 samples, 4 samples are taken from four corners and one from centre.

4. Dissolve 1 g of each sample in 10 ml of water and titration of these samples is done with standard sodium hydroxide solution and takes the reading of sodium hydroxide solution consumed.

5. Repeat the same procedure for 5 samples of brick powder and oxalic acid after mixing 15 minutes in the mixer.

Observation

Weight of oxalic acid + weighing bottle = (w_1)

Weight of oxalic acid + weighing bottle (after removal of oxalic acid) = (w_2)

Weight of oxalic acid (w) = $w_1 - w_2$

$$\text{Normality of oxalic acid} = \frac{1000 \times w}{\text{Equivalent wt.} \times \text{Vol. prepared}}$$

Sr. No.	Volume of oxalic acid (ml)	Burette reading		Volume of sodium hydroxide used (ml)
		Initial	Final	
1.				
2.				
3.				

Normality of NaOH = $N_{NaOH} \times V_{NaOH} = N_{OA} \times V_{OA}$

Sr. No	Weight of sample taken (g)	Duration of mixing (minutes)	Volume of sodium hydroxide used (ml)
1.			
2.			
3.			
4.			
5.			

Calculation

Calculation for samples taken after 5 min of mixing

(a) For sample No. 1- Weight of oxalic acid (C_{A1}) =

(b) For sample No. 2- Weight of oxalic acid (C_{A2}) =

(c) For sample No. 3- Weight of oxalic acid (C_{A3}) =

(d) For sample No. 4- Weight of oxalic acid (C_{A4}) =

(e) For sample No. 5- Weight of oxalic acid (C_{A5}) =

$$C_{MA} = \frac{C_{A1} + C_{A2} + C_{A3} + C_{A4} + C_{A5}}{\eta}$$

where

C_{MA} = Average composition of oxalic acid in mixture

η = No. of samples

C_{A} = Composition of components in single sample

$$\text{Mixing Index } (I_1) = \left[\frac{\Sigma (C_A - C_{MA})^2}{\eta (1 - C_{MA}) C_{MA}} \right]^{0.5}$$

Same procedure is followed for 15 minutes of mixing to get Mixing Index.

Average Mixing Index $(I) = I_1 + I_2$

Result

The Average Mixing Index for given sample was found to be ....

Conclusion

Higher the speed of rotation of mixer, higher will be the efficiency of the mixing.

GLOSSARY

Aromatic water	A clear, saturated aqueous solution of volatile oils or other aromatic or volatile substances.
Bulk powder	A powder which is dispensed in bulk when accuracy of dosage is not critical. Bulk oral powders are limited to relatively non-potent drugs such as laxatives, antacids, dietary supplements, etc.
Dusting powder	A preparation consisting of finely divided powder that is intended to be applied to the skin for therapeutic, prophylactic or lubricant purposes.
Divided powder	A unit dose powder normally packed in properly folded paper and dispensed in envelopes, metal foil, or other suitable containers.
Drops	A liquid preparation in which the quantity to be used at any one time is so small that it is measured as a number of drops. Drops may comprise an oral preparation (usually pediatric) or may be intended for introduction into the nose, ear or eye; the title of the product is amended accordingly.
Elixir	An aromatic liquid preparation including a high proportion of alcohol, glycerin, propylene glycol or other solvent, and intended for the oral administration of potent or nauseous medicaments, in a small dose volume.
Glycerites	A fluid extract of an herb or other medicinal substance made using glycerin as being integral to the fluid extraction medium in not less than 50% by weight of glycerin.
Hydrotrophy	It denotes an increase in solubility of a drug in aqueous medium due to the presence of large amount of additives.

Inhalation	A solution or suspension of one or more drug substances administered to the nasal or oral respiratory route for local or systemic effects. The active principle may be vapor when it is obtained from a liquid preparation by volatilization, or it may be a solid where a special appliance, often an aerosol, is needed.
Insufflations	These are finely divided powders intended for introduction into body cavities such as nose, ears, vagina with the help of insufflators.
Levigation	This is the term applied to the incorporation into the base, of insoluble coarse powders. It is often termed 'wet grinding'. It is the process where the powder is rubbed down with either the molten base or semi-solid base. A considerable shearing force is applied to avoid a gritty product.
Liniment	A liquid or semi-liquid intended for application to intact skin, usually with considerable friction produced by massaging with the hand.
Lotion	A liquid preparation intended for application to the skin without friction.
Lozenge	A solid oral preparation consisting of medicaments incorporated in a flavored base and intended to dissolve or disintegrate slowly in the mouth.
Mucilages	These are thick, viscid, adhesive liquids, produced by dispersing gum in water, or by extracting the mucilaginous ingredients from vegetable substances with water.
Pastille	A solid oral preparation consisting of one or more medicaments in an inert base and intended to dissolve slowly in the mouth.
Pill	A solid oral dose form consisting of one or more medicaments incorporated in a spherical or ovoid mass.
Poultice	A soft, viscous, paste like wet masses of medicament and other solid ingredients applied to the skin while hot to reduce the inflammation, pain or to act as counter-irritant. It is also known as cataplasms.
Powders	A preparation consisting of one or more components in fine powder. It may be in bulk form or individually wrapped quantities and is intended for oral administration. The particle size ranges from 0.1 to 10000 μm.

Solubilization	The spontaneous passage of poorly water soluble solute molecules in an aqueous solution of a surfactant in which a thermodynamically stable solution is formed.
Spirit	An alcoholic solution of volatile medicinal substances or flavoring agents.
Syrup	A liquid preparation containing a high proportion of sucrose or other sweetening agent.
Trituration	This is the term applied to the incorporation, into the base, of finely divided insoluble powders or liquids. The powders are placed on the tile and the base is incorporated using the 'doubling up' technique.

Suggested Readings

1. Indian Pharmacopoeia.

2. British Pharmacopoeia.

3. United States Pharmacopoeia.

4. British Pharmaceutical Codex.

5. N. K. Jain & S.N. Sharma, Text Book of Professional Pharmacy, CBS Publishers & Distributors, New Delhi.

6. N.K. Jain & G.D. Gupta, Modern Dispensing Pharmacy, PharmaMed Press, Hyderabad.

7. Aulton, M.E., Pharmaceutics: The science of doses forms design, Churchill Livingstone, London.

8. Allen, L.V., Popovich, N.G., Ansel, H.C., Ansel's Pharmaceutical Dosage Forms and Drug Delivery Systems, Lippincott Williams and Wilkins.

9. Carter, S.J., Cooper and Gunn's Tutorial Pharmacy, CBS Publishers and Distributors, New Delhi.

10. Gennaro, A.R., Remington: The Science and Practice of Pharmacy, Lippincott Williams and Wilkins.

11. Lachman, L. & Licberman, H.A., Theory and Practice of Industrial Pharmacy, Varghese publishing house, Bombay.

www.ingramcontent.com/pod-product-compliance
Lightning Source LLC
LaVergne TN
LVHW081924160726
843514LV00005B/918